Neurological Syndromes

J. Gordon Millichap

Neurological Syndromes

A Clinical Guide to Symptoms and Diagnosis

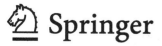 Springer

J. Gordon Millichap, MD., FRCP
Professor Emeritus of Pediatrics and Neurology
Northwestern University Feinberg School of Medicine
Chicago, IL, USA

Pediatric Neurologist
Ann & Robert H. Lurie Children's Hospital of Chicago
Chicago, IL, USA

ISBN 978-1-4614-7785-3   ISBN 978-1-4614-7786-0 (eBook)
DOI 10.1007/978-1-4614-7786-0
Springer New York Heidelberg Dordrecht London

Library of Congress Control Number: 2013943276

Printed on acid-free paper

Springer is part of Springer Science+Business Media (www.springer.com)

Preface

"Syndrome" (from the Greek *syndromos*, running together) is defined as a group of symptoms or signs that collectively characterize a disease or disorder. All of us have had the experience of examining a patient with unusual features or a set of symptoms and signs that appear to be related, and yet we are unable to recall the name of the syndrome or complete set of features. Presented recently with a child who had endured multiple operations for the complications of Goldenhar syndrome, I needed a quick reference book to check the complications that might influence the child's response to treatment of his inattention and hyperactive behavior. I learned that cardiac complications were a recognized feature of the syndrome, and the exclusion of a structural heart defect was a necessary prelude to a prescription for stimulant medication.

A search of the literature failed to uncover a current reference compendium on neurological syndromes, and this experience prompted me to compile a list. My aim was to include recognized syndromes having a significant number of neurological characteristics, and especially those designated by an eponym. The search for syndromes began with the perusal of indices of major neurology and pediatric neurology textbooks and board review books. In this compendium, each syndrome is defined, diagnostic characteristics and associated abnormalities are listed, differential diagnosis and genetics are briefly noted, and a short list of references appended. In all cases, an attempt is made to find and list the original reference, as well as the most recent afforded by a search of PubMed. Several sources were culled for the original reference, and these included major, current, and older textbooks of neurology, Whonamedit? dictionary of medical eponyms, and early review publications.

This compendium is intended as a quick reference guide to the better known and some less familiar syndromes of neurological interest. To those readers who can recall the name of a syndrome, the alphabetical presentation should facilitate a review of the major diagnostic characteristics. The original reference is provided for historical interest, and review articles are included to show recent advances in etiology and treatment. The index is arranged in alphabetical order of the named syndromes and also according to the involvement of various organs in addition to the nervous system. The author has attempted to list all syndromes of neurological interest, and apologies are offered for the inadvertent omission of any recognized and eponymous disorder that involves the nervous system.

Chicago, IL, USA   J. Gordon Millichap, MD., FRCP

Contents

A

Aicardi Syndrome – Avellis Syndrome

Aicardi Syndrome
Aicardi-Goutieres Syndrome
Andermann Syndrome
Angelman Syndrome
Anton Syndrome
Apert Syndrome
Avellis Syndrome

J.G. Millichap, *Neurological Syndromes: A Clinical Guide to Symptoms and Diagnosis*, DOI 10.1007/978-1-4614-7786-0_1,
© Springer Science+Business Media New York 2013

Aicardi Syndrome

- Organs Involved
  - Brain and eyes
- Diagnostic Characteristics
  - Agenesis of the corpus callosum
  - Infantile spasms
  - Chorioretinal lacunae
- Associated Abnormalities
  - Microcephaly, heterotopias, polymicrogyria
  - Cerebellar dysgenesis
  - Microphthalmia, coloboma
  - Costovertebral defects
  - Facial asymmetry
  - Intellectual disability, developmental delay, hypotonia
  - Focal seizures
- Differential Diagnosis
  - Aicardi-Goutieres syndrome, an inherited neonatal encephalopathy
  - Andermann syndrome (corpus callosum agenesis, neuropathy)
- Genetics
  - Sporadic, mainly affecting girls; rarely in 47, XXY males
  - X-linked unidentified gene, dominant mutation, usually lethal in boys
- Treatment
  - Long-term management of infantile spasms and other seizures
  - Parental guidance to cope with developmental retardation
- Prognosis
  - Variable, usually poor, dependent on seizure response to treatment

References

Original:
Aicardi J, Lefebvre J. A new syndrome, spasm in flexion, callosal agenesis, ocular abnormalities. Electroencephalogr Clin Neurophysiol 1965;19:609–610.

Reviews and Case Reports:
Aicardi J. Aicardi syndrome. Brain Dev 2005 Apr;27(3):164–171.
Rosser TL, Acosta MT, Packer RJ. Aicardi syndrome: spectrum of disease and long-term prognosis in 77 females. Pediatr Neurol 2002 Nov;27(5):343–346.
Hopkins B, Sutton VR, Lewis RA, Van den Veyver I, Clark G. Neuroimaging aspects of Aicardi syndrome. Am J Med Genet A 2008 Nov 15;146A(22):2871–2878.

Aicardi-Goutieres Syndrome
(alt. Cree encephalitis, pseudo-Torch syndrome, early-onset familial encephalopathy)

- Organs Involved
  - Brain, CSF, skin, and immune system

- Diagnostic Characteristics
  - Brain atrophy, microcephaly
  - Chronic CSF lymphocytosis
  - Basal ganglia calcification

- Associated Abnormalities
  - Autoimmune disorders such as chilblains (pernio)
  - Increased interferon-alpha in CSF

- Differential Diagnosis
  - Congenital viral encephalitis
  - Systemic lupus erythematosus

- Genetics
  - Autosomal recessive leukodystrophy, genetically and phenotypically heterogeneous
  - Mapped to chromosome 3p21, mutations in one of five genes, TREX1, 3 subunits of the ribonuclease H2 enzyme complex, and SAMHD1

- Treatment
  - For autoimmune diseases, management of seizures and spasticity

- Prognosis
  - Rapidly fatal or a vegetative outcome

References

Original:
Aicardi J, Goutieres F. A progressive familial encephalopathy in infancy with calcifications of the basal ganglia and chronic cerebrospinal fluid lymphocytosis. Ann Neuro 1984;15(1):49–54.

Reviews and Case Reports:
Stephenson JB. Aicardi-Goutieres syndrome (AGS). Eur J Paediatr Neurol 2008 Sep;12(5):355–358.
Chahwan C, Chahwan R. Aicardi-Goutieres syndrome: from patients to genes and beyond. Clin Genet 2012 May;81(5):413–420.

Andermann Syndrome

- Organs Involved
  - Corpus callosum, peripheral nerves, anterior horn cells
- Diagnostic Characteristics
  - Agenesis of corpus callosum
  - Intellectual disability
  - Progressive sensorimotor neuropathy
- Associated Abnormalities
  - Paraparesis
  - Areflexia
  - Microcephaly
  - Seizures
  - Optic atrophy
- Genetics
  - Autosomal recessive disorder, mainly in French-Canadian stock from Quebec, Canada
  - Truncating mutations of the KCC3 gene (SLC12A6) associated; occasional missense mutations

References

Original:

Andermann E, Andermann F, Joubert M, Karpati G, Carpenter S, Melanson D. Familial agenesis of the corpus callosum with anterior horn cell disease: A syndrome of mental retardation, areflexia, and paraparesis. Transactions of the American Neurological Association, New York. 1972;97:242–244.

Review and Case Reports:

Uyanik G, Elcioglu N, Penzien J, et al. Novel truncating and missense mutations of the KCC3 gene associated with Andermann syndrome. Neurology 2006 Apr 11;66(7):1044–1048.

Rudnik-Schoneborn S, Hehr U, von Kalle T, Bornemann A, Winkler J, Zerres K. Andermann syndrome can be a phenocopy of hereditary motor and sensory neuropathy – report of a discordant sibship with a compound heterozygous mutation of the KCC3 gene. Neuropediatrics 2009 Jun;40(3):129–133.

Angelman Syndrome
(alt: Happy puppet syndrome)

- Organs Involved
  - Brain, face, eyes, skin

- Diagnostic Characteristics
  - Developmental delay, ataxia
  - Frequent laughter, hand flapping
  - Speech impairment
  - Microcephaly
  - Seizures, abnormal characteristic EEG

- Associated Abnormalities
  - Protruding tongue, drooling, feeding problems, mouthing behaviors
  - Flat occiput, prominent jaw
  - Hypopigmented skin, light hair
  - Strabismus, scoliosis, hyperreflexia, sleep-cycle disorder
  - Fascination with water and crinkly items

- Differential Diagnosis
  - Rett syndrome
  - Prader-Willi syndrome (loss of paternal gene contribution)
  - Lennox-Gastaut syndrome
  - Infantile autism

- Genetics
  - Loss of normal maternal contribution to chromosome 15 by deletion
  - Deficient UBE3A gene expression on chromosome region 15q11-q13

- Treatment
  - Control of seizures and management of behavior, learning, motor impairment, and sleep disturbance. Genetic counseling

- Prognosis
  - Varies with specific genetic mechanism, and with control of seizures and sleep disturbance. Not a degenerative disease. Symptoms change with age

References

Original:
Angelman H. Puppet children: a report of three cases. Dev Med Child Neurol 1965;7(6):681–688.

Reviews and Case Reports:
Williams CA, Beaudet AL, Clayton-Smith J et al. Angelman syndrome 2005: updated consensus for diagnostic criteria. Am J Med Genet 2006;140A(5):413–418.
Boyd SG, Harden A, Patton MA. The EEG in early diagnosis of the Angelman (happy puppet) syndrome. Eur J Pediatr 1988 Jun;147(5):508–513.

A   Aicardi Syndrome – Avellis Syndrome

Anton Syndrome
(alt: Anton-Babinski syndrome)

- Organs Involved
  - Brain, occipital or parieto-occipital lobes, posterior cerebral artery
- Diagnostic Characteristics
  - Blindness of cerebral origin due to arterial infarcts or trauma. Cortical blindness with normal pupillary responses and absence of optic atrophy
  - Denial of blindness (anosognosia) and confabulation
- Associated Abnormalities
  - Hallucinations
  - Visual agnosia (cannot recognize familiar objects by sight)
  - Prosopagnosia (cannot identify faces)
  - Achromatopsia (cannot recognize colors)
  - Alexia (cannot recognize words or letters)
  - Topographic agnosia (cannot identify relation of objects in space)
- Differential Diagnoses
  - Retrobulbar neuritis
  - Migraine
  - Occipital seizure
  - Blackouts
  - Posterior reversible encephalopathy syndrome (e.g. in pre-eclampsia)
  - Hysteria (functional amaurosis)
- Treatment
  - Early diagnosis and treatment of stroke
- Prognosis
  - Varies with cause, severity of occipital infarct or trauma

References

Original:
Anton G: Über die Selbstwahrnehmung der Herderkrankungen des Gehirns durch den Kranken bei Rindenblindheit und Rindentaubheit. Arch Psychiatrie Nervenkrankh 1899; 32:86–127. (cited in Cogan DG, 1966)
Babinski J: Contribution a l'étude des troubles mentaux dans l'hémiplégie organique (anosognosie). Revue Neurol 1914; 27:845–848

Reviews and Case Reports:
Cogan DG. Neurology of the Visual System. Springfield, IL; Charles C Thomas, 1966.
Redlich FC, Dorsey JF. Denial of blindness by patients with cerebral disease. Arch Neurol Psychiat 1945;53:407. (cited in Cogan DG, 1966)
Critchley, Macdonald. Modes of reaction to central blindness. In Critchley M. The Divine Banquet of the Brain, New York, Raven, 1979;p156.
Trifiletti RR, Syed EH, Hayes-Rosen C, Parano E, Pavone P. Anton-Babinski syndrome in a child with early stage adrenoleukodystrophy. Eur J Neurol 2007 Feb;14(2):e11–e12.

Apert Syndrome
(alt: Acrocephalopolysyndactyly)

- Organs Involved
  - Coronal suture of skull, eyes, hands
- Diagnostic Characteristics
  - Coronal suture synostosis
  - Proptosis
  - Syndactyly (spade [mild], mitten [moderate], and rosebud [severe] hand deformity)
- Associated Abnormalities
  - Hearing loss
  - Prognathism, narrow palate, teeth crowding
  - Heart defects (dextrorotation, patent ductus)
  - Tracheoesophageal fistula
  - Pyloric stenosis
  - Polycystic kidneys
  - Hydrocephalus, cerebral malformation
  - Intellectual deficits
- Differential Diagnosis
  - Crouzon, Pfeiffer, Carpenter, and Saethre-Chotzen syndromes
- Genetics
  - Autosomal dominant, paternal specific mutation in the FGFR2 gene
  - Defect on the fibroblast growth factor receptor 2 gene, on chromosome 10
- Treatment
  - Plastic, oral, maxillofacial and syndactyly surgeries
  - Psychological counseling
- Prognosis
  - Secondary revisions of hand surgery for contractures that develop with age

References

Original:

Apert E. De l'acrocephalosyndactylie. Bulletins et memoires de la Societe medicale des hopitaux de Paris. 1906;23:1310. (Cited in a dictionary of medical eponyms)

Reviews and Case Reports:

Moloney DM, Slaney SF, Oldridge M, et al. Exclusive paternal origin of new mutations in Apert syndrome. Nature Genetics 1996;13(1):48–53.

Kaplan LC. Clinical assessment and multispecialty management of Apert syndrome. Clin Plast Surg 1991 Apr;18(2):217–225.

Da Costa AC, Savarirayan R, Wrennall JA, et al. Neuropsychological diversity in Apert syndrome: a comparison of cognitive profiles. Ann Plast Surg 2005 Apr;54(4):450–455.

Avellis Syndrome

- Organs Involved
  - Tegmentum of medulla
- Diagnostic Characteristics
  - Paralysis of soft palate and vocal cords involving Cr Nerve X and nucleus ambiguuus
  - Contralateral hemianesthesia
  - Horner's syndrome sometimes associated
- Causes
  - Occlusion of vertebral artery and infarct
  - Tumor
- Differential Diagnosis
  - Other brainstem syndromes involving the tegmentum of medulla (Jackson and Wallenberg)

References

Original:
Avellis G. Klinische Beitrage zur halbseitigen Kehlkopflahmung. Berliner Klinik 1891;40:1–26.

Review and Case Reports:
Krasnianski M, Neudecker S, Schluter A, Zierz S. Avellis' syndrome in brainstem infarctions. Fortschr Neurol Psychiatr 2003 Dec;71(12):650–653.

B

Balint Syndrome – Burning Feet Syndrome

Balint Syndrome
Bannwarth Syndrome
Bardet-Biedl Syndrome
Bassen-Kornzweig Syndrome
Benedikt Syndrome
Bobble-Head Doll Syndrome
Brainstem Syndromes
Brown-Sequard Syndrome
Brueghel Syndrome
Burning Feet Syndrome

J.G. Millichap, *Neurological Syndromes: A Clinical Guide to Symptoms and Diagnosis*, DOI 10.1007/978-1-4614-7786-0_2,
© Springer Science+Business Media New York 2013

Balint Syndrome
(alt: A disconnection syndrome)

- **Organs Involved**
  - Brain, bilateral parieto-occipital border zones
- **Diagnostic Characteristics**
  - Simultanagnosia (inability to perceive the visual field as a whole)
  - Ocular apraxia (difficulty in fixating the eyes)
  - Optic ataxia (inability to point to a specific object using vision)
- **Associated Abnormalities**
  - Sudden, severe hypotension
  - Multiple bilateral strokes
  - Alzheimer's disease
  - Traumatic brain injury
  - Intracranial tumors
  - Migraine
- **Treatment**
  - Rehabilitation

References

Original:
Balint R. Seelenlahmung des 'Schauena,' optiche Ataxia, raumliche Storung der Aufmerksamkeit. Monatschr Psychiatr Neurol 1909;25:51–81.

Reviews and Case Reports:
Holmes GM. Disturbances of visual orientation. Brit Jrnl Ophthalmol 1918;2:449–468, 506–516.
Husain M, Stein J. Rezso Balint and his most celebrated case. Arch Neurol 1988 Jan;45(1):89–93.
Mendez MF, Turner J, Gilmore GC, Remler B, Tomsak RL. Balint's syndrome in Alzheimer's disease: visuospatial functions. Int J Neurosci 1990 Oct;54(3–4):339–346.
Gillen JA, Dutton GN. Balint's syndrome in a 10-year-old male. Dev Med Child Neurol 2003 May;45(5):349–352.

Bannwarth Syndrome
(alt: Garin-Bujadoux-Bannwarth syndrome; neuroborreliosis)

- ■ Organs Involved
  - • Meninges, CrN VII, peripheral nerves
- ■ Diagnostic Characteristics
  - • Erythema chronicum migrans
  - • Headache, myalgias
  - • Meningismus
  - • CrN VII paresis
  - • Radiculopathy, mononeuritis multiplex
  - • Peripheral neuropathy
- ■ Treatment
  - • Facial palsy: Doxycycline
  - • CNS involvement: IV cephalosporin, penicillin

References

Original:
Garin Ch, Bujadoux A. Paralysie par les Tiques. J Med Lyon 1922;71:765–767.
Bannworth A. Chronische lymphocytare meningitis, entzundliche polyneuritis und rheumatismus. Ein beitrag zum problem allergie und nervensystem. Archiv fur Psychiatrie und Nervenkrankheiten, Berlin 1941;113:284–376.

Review and Case Reports:
Halperin JJ. Nervous system Lyme disease. Infect Dis Clin North Am 2008 Jun;22(2):261–274.
Halperin JJ, Shapiro ED, Logigian E, et al. Practice parameter: treatment of nervous system Lyme disease (an evidence-base review): report of the Quality Standards Subcommittee of the American Academy of Neurology. Neurology 2007 Jul 3;69(1):91–102.

Bardet-Biedl Syndrome
(alt: Laurence-Moon-Biedl-Bardet syndrome)

- ■ Organs Involved
  - • Brain, hands and feet, eyes, genitourinary

- ■ Diagnostic Characteristics
  - • Obesity
  - • Mental and growth retardation, short stature
  - • Retinitis pigmentosa
  - • Polydactyly
  - • Hypogonadism
  - • Renal dysfunction

- ■ Associated Abnormalities
  - • Anosmia
  - • Cardiomyopathy
  - • Behavior and social problems
  - • Diabetes mellitus, diabetes insipidus

- ■ Genetics
  - • A ciliopathy with defects in the cellular ciliary structure related to mutations in the BBS genes
  - • Autosomal recessive inheritance

References

Original:

Bardet G. Sur un syndrome d'obesite infantile avec polydactylie et retinite pigmentaire. Therese de Paris. 1920, No 479.

Biedl A. Ein geschwisterpaar mit adipose-genitaler dystrophie. Deutsche medicinische Wochenschrift, Berlin. 1922;48:1630.

Reviews and Case Reports:

Millichap JG. Laurence-Moon-Biedl syndrome. Proc R Soc Med 1951 Dec;44(12):1063–1064.

Ansley SJ, Badano H, Blacque OE, et al. Basal body dysfunction is a likely cause of pleiotropic Bardet-Biedl syndrome. Nature 2003 Oct;425(6958):628–633.

Lee JE, Gleeson JG. Cilia in the nervous system: linking cilia function and neurodevelopmental disorders. Curr Opin Neurol 2011 Apr;24(2):98–105.

Bassen-Kornzweig Syndrome
(alt: Abetalipoproteinemia)

- Organs Involved
  - Red blood cells, retina, spinal cord and myelinated nerves, intestine
- Diagnostic Characteristics
  - Fat malabsorption
  - Acanthocytosis
  - Retinitis pigmentosa, decreased night vision
  - Vitamin A, D, E, and K deficiency; absent B-lipoproteins; low cholesterol
  - Sensory neuropathy, decreased reflexes and sensation, positive Romberg
  - Spinocerebellar and posterior column degeneration
- Associated Abnormalities
  - Fatty, frothy, foul-smelling stools
  - Failure to thrive in infancy
  - Protruding abdomen
  - Developmental delay, muscle weakness, dyspraxia
  - Slurred speech
  - Scoliosis
  - Visual impairment
  - Progressive ataxia and incoordination
- Differential Diagnosis
  - Friedreich ataxia
  - Friedreich-like ataxia with isolated vitamin E deficiency
- Genetics
  - Autosomal recessive, with mutations in the microsomal triglyceride transfer protein (MTTP) gene, essential for B-lipoprotein production
- Treatment
  - Vitamin E supplements, dietary restriction of triglycerides

References

Original:
Bassen FA, Kornzweig AL. Malformation of erythrocytes in a case of atypical retinitis pigmentosa. Blood 1950;5(4):381–387.

Review and Case Reports:
Stevenson VL, Hardie RJ. Acanthocytosis and neurological disorders. J Neurol 2001 Feb;248(2):87–94.
Chardon L, Sassolas A, Dingeon B, et al. Identification of two novel mutations and long-term follow-up in abetalipoproteinemia: a report of four cases. Eur J Pediatr 2009 Aug;168(8): 983–989.

Benedikt Syndrome
(alt: Paramedian midbrain syndrome)

- Organs Involved
  - Cranial nerve III, red nucleus, midbrain tegmentum, brachium conjunctivum, corticospinal tracts, cerebellum
- Diagnostic Characteristics
  - Ipsilateral oculomotor palsy
  - Contralateral cerebellar ataxia, tremor, and hemiparesis
- Associated Abnormalities
  - Occlusion of posterior cerebral artery or paramedian branches of the basilar artery
  - Infarction, hemorrhage, tumor, or tuberculosis in tegmentum of midbrain and cerebellum
- Differential Diagnosis
  - Weber syndrome
  - Claude syndrome
  - Wallenberg syndrome
- Treatment
  - Deep brain stimulation may relieve tremors
  - Rehabilitation

References

Original:
Benedikt M. Tremeblement avec paralysie croisee du moteur oculaire commun. Bull Med Paris 1889;3:547. (Cited in Garrison's History of Neurology, by McHenry LC, Springfield, IL, Charles C Thomas, 1969)

Review and Case Reports:
Akdal G, Kutluk K, Men S, Yaka E. Benedikt and "plus-minus lid" syndromes arising from posterior cerebral artery branch occlusion. J Neurol Sciences 2005 Jan;228(1):105–107.
Brandt SK, Anderson D, BNiller J. Deep brain stimulation as an effective treatment option for post-midbrain infarction-related tremor as it presents with Benedikt syndrome. Jrnl Neurosurgery 2008 Oct;109(4):635–639.

Bobble-Head Doll Syndrome

- Organs Involved
  - Head and shoulders, third ventricle in brain
- Diagnostic Characteristics
  - Bobbing of head at 2–3 s (side to side, to and fro); average age at onset 3 years (range: infancy to adulthood)
  - Movement stops during mental tasks (e.g., spelling, adding)
  - Movement stops during sleep
  - Third ventricle cystic lesion, choroid plexus papilloma
  - Suprasellar arachnoid cyst
  - Obstruction of foramina of Monro and cerebral aqueduct
  - Hydrocephalus, macrocephaly
- Associated Abnormalities
  - Ataxia
- Treatment
  - Surgical removal of cyst
  - Ventriculoperitoneal shunt
- Prognosis
  - Earlier the treatment, better the prognosis
  - Complete recovery in 50 %

References

Original:

Benton JW, Nellhaus G, Huttenlocher PR, Ojemann RG, Dodge PR. The bobble-head doll syndrome: report of unique truncal tremor associated with third ventricular cyst and hydrocephalus in children. Neurology 1966;16(8):725–729.

Review and Case Reports:

Nellhaus G. Bobble-head doll syndrome – a tic with a neuropathologic basis. Pediatrics 1967 Aug;40(2):250–3.

Wiese JA, Gentry LR, Menezes AH. Bobble-head doll syndrome: review of the pathophysiology and CSF dynamics. Pediatr Neurol 1985;1(6):361–366.

Guerreiro H, Vlasak A, Horinek D, et al. Bobble-head doll syndrome: therapeutic outcome and long-term follow-up in four children. Acta Neurochir (Wien) 2012 Nov;154(11):2043–2049.

Brainstem Syndromes

Eponym	Location	CrN palsy	Crossed tract signs	Cause
Weber	Midbrain	III	Hemiplegia	Stroke, tumor
Claude	Midbrain	III	Cerebellar ataxia	Stroke, tumor
Benedikt	Midbrain	III	Ataxia/hemiplegia	Stroke, tumor
Nothnagel	Midbrain	III	Ataxia	Tumor
Millard-Gubler	Ventral pons	VII, VI	Hemiplegia	Infarct, tumor
Foville	Dorsal pons	VII, VI	Hemiplegia	Infarct, tumor
Avellis	Medulla	X palate/vocal	Hemianesthesia	Infarct, tumor
Jackson	Medulla	X, XII tongue	Hemianesthesia	Infarct, tumor
Wallenberg	Lateral medulla	Spnl V, IX, X, XI	Loss of pain/temperature	PICA infarct

Abbreviated and modified from Table 34.3 in Adams and Victor's Principles of Neurology, Ninth Edition, Ropper AH, Samuels MA, eds. New York, McGraw-Hill Companies, 2009. p764. See also individual alphabetical syndrome entries

Brown-Sequard Syndrome
(alt: Crossed hemiplegia)

- Organs Involved
  - Spinal cord, corticospinal tract, dorsal column, spinothalamic tract
- Diagnostic Characteristics
  - Ipsilateral spastic paralysis below the lesion
  - Ipsilateral loss of light touch, vibration, and position sense
  - Contralateral loss of pain and temperature sensation
- Causes
  - Gunshot or knife puncture wound to neck or back
  - Ischemia, vascular infarct of sulco-commissural artery
  - Inflammatory or infectious, multiple sclerosis or tuberculosis
  - Spinal tumor

References

Original:

Brown-Sequard CE. De la transmission croisee des impressions sensitives par la moelle epiniere. Comptes rendus de la Societe de biologie. 1850;2:33–44.

Reviews and Case Reports:

Millichap JJ, Sy BT, Leacock RO. Spinal cord infarction with multiple etiologic factors. J Gen Intern Med 2007 Jan;22(1):151–154.

Lim E, Wong YS, Lo YL, Lim SH. Traumatic atypical Brown-Sequard syndrome: case report and literature review. Clin Neurol Neurosurg 2003 April;105(2):143–145.

Kraus JA, Stuper BK, Berlit P. Multiple sclerosis presenting with a Brown-Sequard syndrome. J Neurol Sci 1998;156(1):112–113.

Sayer FT, Vitali AM, Low HL, Paquette S, Honey CR. Brown-Sequard syndrome produced by C3-C4 cervical disc herniation: a case report and review of the literature. Spine (Phila Pa 1976) 2008 Apr 20;33(9):E279–82.

Brueghel Syndrome
(alt: Meige syndrome, oral facial dystonia)

- Organs Involved
  - Face, jaw
- Diagnostic Characteristics
  - Oromandibular dystonia – chin thrusting, trismus, bruxism, lip pursing, tongue protrusion, dysphagia, dysarthria
  - Blepharospasm symptoms – involuntary increased blinking, squinting, photophobia, uncontrolled eye closure
  - Onset between 30 and 70 years of age; women to men ratio 2:1
- Additional Abnormalities
  - Spasmodic dysphonia, spasmodic torticollis, laryngeal dystonia
  - Dystonic spasms may be provoked by talking, chewing, or biting
- Treatment
  - Botox injections
  - Surgery – deep brain stimulation of globus pallidus internus

References

Original:
Meige H. Les convulsions de la face, une forme clinique de convulsion faciale, bilaterale et mediane. Revue Neurologique, Paris. 1910;20:437–443.
Marsden CD. Blepharospasm-oromandibular dystonia syndrome (Brueghel's syndrome). A variant of adult-onset torsion dystonia. Jrnl Neurol, Neurosurgery and Psychiatry, London. 1976;39:1204–1209.

Review and Case Reports:
Reese R, Gruber D, Schoenecker T, et al. Long-term clinical outcome in meige syndrome treated with internal pallidum deep brain stimulation. Mov Disord 2011 Mar;26(4):691–698.
Miyaoka T, Miura S, Seno H, Inagaki T, Horiguchi J. Jaw-opening dystonia (Brueghel's syndrome) associated with cavum septi pellucidi and Verga's ventricle – a case report. Eur J Neurol 2003 Nov;10(6):727–729.

Burning Feet Syndrome
(alt: Chronic mild sensory polyneuropathy of the elderly)
(Grierson and Gopalan syndrome)

- ■ Organs Involved
  - • Small unmyelinated C-fiber peripheral nerves, autonomic nervous system

- ■ Diagnostic Characteristics
  - • Small fiber neuropathy, especially in the elderly
  - • Painful burning sensations in the feet (slowly progressive over years)
  - • Paresthesias and hyperesthesia in feet, ankles, and lower legs
  - • Normal motor and sensory examination (mild ataxia in some)

- ■ Etiology
  - • Idiopathic (of elderly)
  - • Nutritional, vitamin B deficiencies
  - • Metabolic, diabetic neuropathy; endocrine, hypothyroidism
  - • Entrapment and compression of peripheral nerves in spine (spinal stenosis) or peripherally as in tarsal tunnel syndrome
  - • Genetic, dominantly inherited in rare cases

- ■ Diagnostic Tests
  - • Skin biopsy, evaluation of density of intraepidermal nerve fibers
  - • Tests of autonomic nerve function
  - • Metabolic for diabetes, and serum levels of B vitamins
  - • MRI lumbosacral spine

- ■ Treatment
  - • Varies with etiology: physiotherapy, NSAIDs, gabapentin, foot creams
  - • Specific if nutritional, metabolic, or endocrine; surgical decompression

References

Original:
Grierson J. On the burning feet of natives. Transactions of the Medical and Physical Society of Calcutta 1826;2:275–280.
Gopalan C. The "burning feet syndrome." Indian Medical Gazette, Calcutta. 1946;81:22–26. JAMA 1946;131:1177.

Review:
Makkar RPS, Arora A, Monga A, Gupta AK, Mukhopadhyay S. Burning feet syndrome. A clinical review. Australian Family Physician 2002 Dec;31(12):1006–1009.
Tavee J, Zhou L Small fiber neuropathy: A burning problem. Cleve Clin J Med 2009 May;76(5): 297–305.
Dyck PJ, Low PA, Stevens JC. Burning feet as the only manifestation of dominantly inherited sensory neuropathy. Mayo Clin Proc 1983;58(7):426–429.
Ropper AH, Samuels MA eds. Diseases of the Peripheral Nerves. In: Adams and Victor's Principles of Neurology. New York, McGraw Hill, 2009; Chap 46;1296–7.

C

CADASIL Syndrome – Crouzon Syndrome

CADASIL Syndrome
Capgras Syndrome
Cayler Cardiofacial Syndrome
Central Cord Syndrome
CHARGE Syndrome
Charles Bonnet Syndrome (CBS)
Chiasmal Syndrome (Junctional Scotoma Syndrome)
Churg-Strauss Syndrome
Claude Syndrome
Cockayne Syndrome
Coffin-Lowry Syndrome
Cohen Syndrome
Cornelia de Lange Syndrome
Cornelia de Lange Syndrome II
Costen Syndrome
Cowden Syndrome
Cranial Nerve Syndromes
CRASH Syndrome
Cri du Chat Syndrome
Crouzon Syndrome

J.G. Millichap, *Neurological Syndromes: A Clinical Guide to Symptoms and Diagnosis*, DOI 10.1007/978-1-4614-7786-0_3,
© Springer Science+Business Media New York 2013

CADASIL Syndrome
(alt: Cerebral autosomal dominant arteriopathy with subcortical infarcts and leukoencephalopathy)

- Organs Involved
  - Brain arteries and arterioles
- Diagnostic Characteristics
  - Migraine headaches
  - Transient ischemic attacks or stroke; a hereditary stroke disorder
  - Age of onset 40–50 years
  - Leukoencephalopathy
  - Progression to subcortical dementia
- Associated Abnormalities
  - Pseudobulbar palsy
  - Lacunar infarcts
  - Deposition of granular material in the media of small arteries and arterioles
  - Cognitive impairment
- Diagnosis
  - MRI hypointensities on T1-weighted images and hyperintensities on T2-weighted images of anterior temporal lobes; multiple white matter lesions around the basal ganglia, periventricular white matter, and pons
- Genetics
  - Autosomal dominant inheritance
  - Mutations in the Notch 3 gene, on chromosome 19
- Differential Diagnosis
  - CARASIL (Maeda syndrome), a cerebral autosomal recessive arteriopathy with subcortical infarcts and leukoencephalopathy

References

Original:
Joutel A, Corpechot CV, Ducros A, et al. Notch3 mutations in CADASIL, a hereditary adult-onset condition causing stroke and dementia. Nature 1996 Oct;383(6602):707–710.
Chabriat H, Vahedi K, Iba-Zizen MT, et al. Clinical spectrum of CADASIL: a study of 7 families. Cerebral autosomal dominant arteriopathy with subcortical infarcts and leukoencephalopathy. Lancet 1995 Oct;346(8980):934–939.

Review and Case Reports:
Arima K, Yanagawa S, Ito N, Ikeda S. Cerebral arterial pathology of CADASIL and CARASIL (Maeda syndrome). Neuropathology 2003 Dec;23(4):327–334.

Capgras Syndrome
(alt: Capgras delusional misidentification syndrome)

- ■ Organs Involved
  - • Brain and face

- ■ Diagnostic Characteristics
  - • The delusion that a close relative or friend has been replaced by an identical-looking imposter
  - • Misidentification of people, places, or objects
  - • Acute, transient, or chronic disorder

- ■ Associated Abnormalities
  - • Schizophrenia, brain injury, dementia, neurodegenerative disease
  - • Involvement of frontal lobe. Some argue a disconnection between temporal lobe cortex (face recognition) and the limbic system (emotion)
  - • May occur in association with diabetes, hypothyroidism, and migraine
  - • May be induced by some drugs (ketamine)

- ■ Gender Frequencies
  - • More frequent in females; female: male ratio of 3:2

- ■ Differential Diagnosis
  - • Prosopagnosia (inability to recognize familiar faces); involvement of bilateral inferior occipitotemporal region

- ■ Treatment
  - • Cognitive behavioral therapy
  - • Antipsychotic drugs

References

Original:
Capgras J, Reboul-Lachaux J. L'illusion des 'sosies' dans un delire systematise chronique. Bull Soc Clinique Med Mentale. 1923;2:6–16.

Reviews and Case Reports:
Dohn HH, Crews EL. Capgras syndrome: a literature review and case series. Hillside J Clin Psychiatry 1986;8(1):56–74.
Förstl H, Almeida OP, Owen A, Burns A, Howard R. Psychiatric, neurological and medical aspects of misidentification syndromes: a review of 260 cases. Psychol Med 1991 Nov;21(4):905–910.

Cayler Cardiofacial Syndrome
(alt: Asymmetric crying facies)

- Organs Involved
  - Heart and face
- Diagnostic Characteristics
  - Asymmetry of face when crying
  - Unilateral facial weakness (left side in 80 % cases)
  - Hypoplasia of depressor anguli oris muscle
  - Congenital cardiac defects
- Associated Abnormalities
  - Other birth defects in 50 % cases
  - Micrognathia, microphthalmia, microcephaly
  - Genitourinary abnormalities
  - ADHD, autism, mental retardation
  - Neonatal vasomotor instability
- Differential Diagnosis
  - Cranial VII nerve palsy
  - Other 22q11.2 deletion syndromes (e.g., DiGeorge syndrome)
- Genetics
  - Chromosome 22q11.2 deletion
  - Sporadic, sometimes autosomal dominant
- Treatment
  - Correction of associated abnormalities
- Prognosis
  - Variable with degree of incapacity

References

Original:
Cayler GG. Cardiofacial syndrome. Congenital heart disease and facial weakness, a hitherto
   unrecognized association. Arch Dis Child 1969;44:69–75.

Review and Case Reports:
Lahat E, Heyman E, Barkay A, Goldberg M. Asymmetric crying facies and associated congenital
   anomalies: prospective study and review of the literature. J Child Neurol 2000;15(12):808–810.

Central Cord Syndrome
(alt: Schneider syndrome)

- Organs Involved
  - Cervical spinal cord

- Diagnostic Characteristics
  - Acute cervical spinal cord injury with incomplete paralysis
  - Greater motor loss in upper extremities compared to lower
  - Sensory impairment below level of injury
  - Bladder dysfunction and urinary retention

- Causes
  - Occurs with spinal hyperextension injury in older individual with cervical spondylosis
  - May occur with trauma and/or bleeding in central part of cord in younger individuals
  - Complication of generalized tonic-clonic seizure or status epilepticus

- Prognosis
  - Generally favorable for some degree of recovery, dependent on age and extent of injury

References

Original:

Schneider RC, Cherry G, Pantek H. The syndrome of acute central cervical spinal cord injury; with special reference to the mechanisms involved in hyperextension injuries of cervical spine. J Neurosurg 1954;11(6):546–577.

Review and Case Reports:

Lee S, Lee JE, Yang S, Chang H. A case of central cord syndrome related status epilepticus – a case report-. Ann Rehabil Med 2011 Aug;35(4):574–578.

Yadla S, Klimo P, Harrop JS. Traumatic central cord syndrome: etiology, management, and outcomes. Topics in Spinal Cord Injury Rehabilitation 2010;15(3):73–84.

CHARGE Syndrome

- Organs Involved
  - Eye, heart, nose, brain, genitals, and ear
- Diagnostic Characteristics
  - *C*: Coloboma
  - *H*: Congenital *h*eart defect
  - *A*: Choanal *a*tresia
  - *R*: Mental *r*etardation
  - *G*: Microgenitalia
  - *E*: *E*ar deformity
- Associated Abnormalities
  - Visual impairment
  - Circulation, breathing, and swallowing problems
  - Learning difficulties
  - Hypospadias, undescended testicles
  - Deafness
  - Leading cause of congenital deaf/blindness
- Genetics
  - Autosomal dominant
  - Mutations on the CHD7 gene in 60 % cases. Chromosome 8
- Treatment
  - Airway stabilization and gastrostomy tube installation
  - Cardiac consultation, circulatory support
  - Speech and deaf/blind support, special education
- Prognosis
  - 70 % survival to 5 years of age. Highest mortality in first year
  - High postoperative mortality. Difficult intubation

References

Original:
Hall BD. Choanal atresia and associated multiple anomalies. J Pediatr 1979;95(3):395–398.
Hittner HM, Hirsch NJ, Kreh GM, Rudolph AJ. Colobomatous microphthalmia, heart disease, hearing loss, and mental retardation—a syndrome. J Pediatr Ophthalmology and Strabismus 1979;16(2):122–128.
Pagan RA, Graham JM, Zonana J, Young SL. Coloboma, congenital heart disease, and choanal atresia with multiple anomalies: CHARGE association. J Pediatr 1981;99(2):223–227.

Review, Genetics, and Case Reports:
Lalani SR, Safiullah AM, Fernbach SD, et al. Spectrum of CHD7 mutations in 110 individuals with CHARGE syndrome and genotype-phenotype correlation. Am J Hum Genet 2006;78(2):303–314.

Charles Bonnet Syndrome (CBS)

- Organs Involved
  - Eyes, visual pathways, and cortex
- Diagnostic Characteristics
  - Visual impairment, often in psychologically normal elderly population
  - Complex recurrent visual hallucinations, lilliputian cartoons of men, women, birds, buildings, tapestries, and scaffolding patterns
  - Patient is aware that the hallucination is not real
  - Prevalence varies from 10 % to 40 % in elderly with visual loss
- Associated Abnormalities
  - Cataracts, macular degeneration
  - Occipital lobe seizures
  - Viral encephalitis
  - Pituitary tumor
- Prognosis
  - Last a few seconds to all day, 1 year to 18 months intermittently
- Treatment
  - Any underlying illness

References

Original:

Bonnet C. Essai analytique sur les faculties de l'ame. 1st edition, Copenhagen 1760; 2nd edition, Copenhagen 1769;vol 2:176–178.

Review and Case Reports:

Tan C, Lim V, Ho D, Yeo E, Ng B, Au Eong E. Charles Bonnet syndrome in Asian patients in a tertiary ophthalmic center. Brit J Ophthalmol 2005;88(10):1325–1329.

Aydin OF, Ince H, Tasdemir HA, Ozyurek H. Charles Bonnet syndrome after herpes simplex encephalitis. Pediatr Neurol 2012 Apr;46(4):250–252.

Brown-Vargas D, Cienki JJ. Occipital lobe epilepsy presenting as Charles Bonnet syndrome. Am J Emerg Med 2012 Nov;30(9):2102.e-5–6.

Chiasmal Syndrome
(Junctional Scotoma Syndrome)

- ■ Organs Involved
  - • Optic chiasm
- ■ Diagnostic Characteristics
  - • Anterior chiasmal lesion:
  - • Ipsilateral junctional central scotoma with optic disc neuropathy
  - • Contralateral superotemporal field defect
  - • Middle lesion affecting crossing nasal retinal fibers:
  - • Bitemporal hemianopia
  - • Posterior chiasmal syndrome:
  - • Macular fiber damage, smaller paracentral bitemporal field loss
- ■ Associated Abnormalities
  - • Optic disc pallor
  - • Hydrocephalus, compression of 3rd ventricle
  - • Hypopituitarism
- ■ Etiology
  - • Intrinsic lesions: gliomas with neurofibromatosis type 1, multiple sclerosis
  - • Extrinsic compressive: pituitary adenoma, craniopharyngioma, meningioma
  - • Metabolic, toxic, traumatic, infectious
  - • Pituitary tumors are most common cause of chiasmal syndrome
  - • Cushing's syndrome, galactorrhea, acromegaly
  - • Pituitary apoplexy with hemorrhagic adenoma
- ■ Management
  - • MRI and endocrine panel

References

Foroozan R. Chiasmal syndromes. Curr Opin Ophthalmol 2003 Dec;14(6):325–331.

Mojon DS, Odel JG, Rios RJ, Hirano M. Pituitary adenoma revealed by paracentral junctional scotoma of traquair. Ophthalmologica 1997;211(2):104–108.

Liu A, Chen YW, Chang S, Liao YJ. Junctional visual field loss in a case of Wyburn-Mason syndrome. J Neuroophthalmol 2012 Mar;32(1):42–44.

Churg-Strauss Syndrome
(alt: Churg-Strauss vasculitis)

- Organs Involved
  - Medium and small arteries, lungs, gastrointestines, peripheral nerves, heart, skin, kidneys, central nervous system

- Diagnostic Characteristics
  - Onset with allergic rhinitis and asthma-like respiratory symptoms
  - Vasculitis involving small and medium arteries and multiple organs
  - Mono- or polyneuropathy
  - Blood eosinophilia >10 %
  - Pulmonary infiltrates

- Associated Abnormalities
  - Eosinophilic granulocytes and granulomas
  - Antineutrophil cytoplasmic antibodies (ANCA)
  - Cerebral infarction

- Treatment
  - Prednisolone, azathioprine, cyclophosphamide

- Prognosis
  - Disease is chronic and lifelong.

References

Original:
Churg J, Strauss L. Allergic granulomatosis, allergic angiitis, and periarteritis nodosa. Am J Pathol 1951;27(2):277–301.

Reviews and Case Reports:
Sehgal M, Swanson JW, DeRemee RA, Colby TV. Neurologic manifestations of Churg-Strauss syndrome. Mayo Clin Proc 1995 Apr;70(4):337–341.
Wolf J, Bergner R, Mutallib S, Buggle F, Grau AJ. Neurologic complications of Churg-Strauss syndrome-a prospective monocentric study. Eur J Neurol 2010 Apr;17(4):582–588.

Claude Syndrome

- ■ Organs Involved
  - • Tegmentum of midbrain
  - • Cranial N III
  - • Red nucleus and brachium conjunctivum
- ■ Diagnostic Characteristics
  - • Ipsilateral oculomotor palsy
  - • Contralateral cerebellar ataxia and tremor
- ■ Causes
  - • Vascular occlusion, branch of posterior cerebral artery
  - • Tumor
- ■ Differential Diagnosis
  - • Other intramedullary brainstem syndromes (Weber, Benedikt, Nothnagel, Millard-Gubler, Parinaud, Avellis, Jackson, Wallenberg)

References

Original:
Claude H, Loyez M. Ramollissement du noyau rouge. Rev Neurol (Paris) 1912;24:49–51

Review and Case Reports:
Seo SW, Heo JH, Lee KY, et al. Localization of Claude's syndrome. Neurology 2001 Dec 26;57(12):2304–2307

Cockayne Syndrome
(alt: Cerebro-oculo-facio-skeletal syndrome, type II CS)

- ■ Organs Involved
  - Eye, ear, nervous system, skeleton

- ■ Diagnostic Characteristics
  - Impaired vision and sensorineural deafness
  - Progressive central and peripheral nervous system degeneration
  - Dwarfism, progeria, contractures
  - Photosensitive skin

- ■ Associated Abnormalities
  - Retinitis pigmentosa, cataracts
  - Mental retardation
  - Basal ganglia calcifications, patchy demyelination
  - Peripheral neuropathy
  - Sudanophilic leukodystrophy with cerebellar ataxia and nystagmus
  - Xeroderma pigmentosum sometimes associated

- ■ Genetics
  - Autosomal recessive congenital disorder. Mutations in the ERCC6 gene account for ~70 % cases; ERCC8 involved in remainder
  - Types I, II, and III. Defect in DNA repair mechanism

- ■ Prognosis
  - Type I has onset in the first 2 years life, and life span is 10–20 years.
  - Type II onset at birth and death by age 7.
  - Type III rare, late onset, and milder than types I and II.

References

Original:
Cockayne EA. Dwarfism with retinal atrophy and deafness. Arch Dis Child 1936;21:53–4

Review and Case Reports:
Nance MA, Berry SA. Cockayne syndrome: review of 140 cases. Am J Med Genet 1992;42:68–84.
Rapin I, Lindenbaum Y, Dickson DW, Kraemer KH, Robbins JH. Cockayne syndrome and xeroderma pigmentosum: DNA repair disorders with overlaps and paradoxes. Neurology 2000 Nov 28;55(10):1442–1449.

Coffin-Lowry Syndrome

- Organs Involved
  - Brain, face, spine, limbs
- Diagnostic Characteristics
  - Severe mental retardation
  - Retarded growth and dwarfism
  - Kyphoscoliosis
  - Tapering fingers
  - Micrognathia, maxillary hypoplasia
  - Prominent brow, hypertelorism, bushy eyebrows
  - Hearing impairment
  - Paroxysmal stimulus-induced, nonepileptic, drop episodes
- Genetics
  - X-linked dominant inheritance
  - Mutations in the RPS6KA3 gene, located on the short arm of the X chromosome (Xp22.2)
- Treatment
  - Symptomatic only
  - Drop attacks fail to respond to antiepileptic drugs, but may respond to sodium oxybate

References

Original:
Coffin GS, Siris E, Wegienka LC. Mental retardation with osteocartilaginous anomalies. Am J Dis Children, Chicago 1966;112:205–213.
Lowry RB, Miller JR, Fraser FC. A new dominant gene mental retardation syndrome: associated with small stature, tapering fingers, characteristic facies, and possible hydrocephalus. Am J Dis Children, Chicago 1971;121:496–500.

Review and Case Reports:
Kesler SR, Simensen RJ, Voeller K, et al. Altered neurodevelopment associated with mutations of RSK2: a morphometric MRI study of Coffin-Lowry syndrome. Neurogenetics 2007 Apr;8(2):143–147.
Havaligi N, Matadeen-Ali C, Khurana DS, Marks H, Kothare SV. Treatment of drop attacks in Coffin-Lowry syndrome with the use of sodium oxybate. Pediatr Neurol 2007 Nov;37(5): 373–374.
Hahn JS, Hanauer A. Stimulus-induced drop episodes in Coffin-Lowry syndrome. Eur J Med Genet 2012 May;55(5):335–337.

Cohen Syndrome
(alt: Pepper syndrome; Cervenka syndrome)

- Organs Involved
  - Brain, head, face, teeth, limbs

- Diagnostic Characteristics
  - Developmental delay, mental retardation
  - Microcephaly
  - Obesity with thin/elongated limbs
  - Craniofacial dysmorphism: micrognathia, thick hair and eyebrows, long eyelashes, downslanting eyes, bulbous nose, short philtrum, prominent upper incisors, open mouth appearance, periodontal disease
  - Hypotonia, hypermobility of joints, motor clumsiness
  - Ocular abnormalities: optic atrophy, microphthalmia, chorioretinitis, hemeralopia, strabismus, nystagmus, coloboma

- Associated Abnormalities
  - Clinical heterogeneity
  - Granulocytopenia
  - Seizures
  - MRI brain enlarged corpus callosum

- Genetics
  - Inherited in autosomal recessive pattern with variable expression
  - Mutations in the COH1 (VPS13B) gene on chromosome 8 at locus 8q22

References

Original:
Cohen MM Jr, Hall BD, Smith DW. A new syndrome with hypotonia, obesity, mental deficiency, and oral, ocular and limb anomalies. J Pediatr 1973;83:280–284.

Reviews and Case Reports:
Carey JC, Hall BD. Confirmation of the Cohen syndrome. J Pediatr 1978 Aug;93(2):239–244.
Kivitie-Kallio S, Norio R. Cohen syndrome: essential features, natural history, and heterogeneity. Am J Med Genet 2001 Aug 1;102(2):125–135.
Douzgou S, Petersen MB. Clinical variability of genetic isolates of Cohen syndrome. Clin Genet 2011 Jun;79(6):501–506.

Cornelia de Lange Syndrome
(alt: Bushy syndrome; Amsterdam dwarfism)

- Organs Involved
  - Face, hair, hands and feet, intestine, heart, brain, genitalia
- Diagnostic Characteristics
  - Low birth weight, short stature, developmental delay
  - Microcephaly, missing limbs, small hands and feet
  - Bushy joined eyebrows (synophrys), long eyelashes, excessive body hair
  - Behavior problems, self-stimulation, aggression, autistic like
  - Gastrointestinal disorders
  - Seizures
  - Heart defects
  - Large genitalia
- Genetics
  - Multiple genes (CDLS1-3) involved on chromosomes 5, X, and 10
  - Majority due to spontaneous mutations

References

Original:
De Lange C. Sur un type nouveau de degeneration (typus Amstelodamensis). Arch Med Enfants 1933;36:713–719.
Opitz JM. The Brachmann-de Lange syndrome. Am J Med Genet, New York 1985;22:89–102.

Review and Case Reports:
Schrier SA, Sherer I, Deardorff MA, et al. Causes of death and autopsy findings in a large study cohort of individuals with Cornelia de Lange syndrome and review of the literature. Am J Med Genet A 2011 Dec;155A(12):3007–3024.
Deardorff MA, Clark DM, Krantz ID. Cornelia de Lange syndrome. In: Pagon RA, Bird TD, Dolan CR, Stephens K, Adam MP, editors. GeneReviews [Internet], Seattle (WA): University of Washington, Seattle, 1993–2005 Sep 16 [updated 2011 Oct 27].

Cornelia de Lange Syndrome II
(alt: Bruck-de Lange syndrome)

- Organs Involved
  - Muscles, neck, extremities, head, brain, heart, intestines
- Diagnostic Characteristics
  - Congenital hypertrophy of muscles, hypertonia, thick neck
  - Extrapyramidal disorders
  - Short, thick extremities
  - Asymmetrical skull, large ears and tongue
  - Porencephaly, large ventricles, large vermis
  - Status spongiosus
  - Small heart
  - Severe mental and motor retardation
- Prognosis
  - Life span < 2 years
  - Familial tendency, mostly sporadic

References

Original:

De Lange C. Congenital hypertrophy of the muscles, extrapyramidal motor disturbances and mental deficiency. A clinical study. Am J Dis Children, Chicago 1934;48:243–268.

Bruck F. Uber einen fall von congenitaler macroglossie, kombiniert mit aligemeiner wahrer muskelhypertrophie und idiotie. Deutsche medicinische Wochenschrift, Berlin 1889;15:229–232.

Review and Case Reports:

Ptacek LJ, Opitz JM, Smith DW, Gerritsen T, Waisman HA. The Cornelia de Lange syndrome. J Pediatr 1963 Nov;63:1000–1020.

Kline AD, Krantz ID, Sommer A, et al. Cornelia de Lange syndrome: clinical review, diagnostic and scoring systems, and anticipatory guidance. Am J Med Genet A 2007 Jun 15;143A(12): 1287–1296.

Costen Syndrome
(alt: Temporomandibular joint disorder; TMJ syndrome;
TMJ pain-dysfunction syndrome)

- Organs Involved
  - Temporomandibular joint, oral musculoskeletal system
- Diagnostic Characteristics
  - Acute or chronic pain in muscles of mastication and/or inflammation of temporomandibular joint
  - Bruxism
  - Biting or chewing discomfort
  - Dull, aching pain in face and jaw
  - Earache (in the morning), tinnitus, hearing loss
  - Migraine headache (in the morning)
- Causes
  - Bruxism
  - Over-opening of jaw
  - Mal-aligned teeth

References

Original:
Costen JB. A syndrome of ear and sinus symptoms dependent upon disturbed function of the temporomandibular joint. Annals of Otology, Rhinology and Laryngology, St Louis 1934;43: 1–15.
Costen JB. Neuralgias and ear symptoms associated with disturbed function of the temporomandibular joint. JAMA 1936;107:252.

Review and Case Reports:
Reik L, Hale M. The temporomandibular joint pain-dysfunction syndrome: A frequent cause of headache. Headache: The Journal of Head and Face Pain 1981;21:151–156.

Cowden Syndrome
(alt: Multiple hamartomas syndrome)

- Organs Involved
  - Skull, skin, intestine, cerebellum, and others
- Diagnostic Characteristics
  - Macrocephaly
  - Intestinal hamartomatous polyps
  - Benign skin tumors
  - Dysplastic gangliocytoma of the cerebellum (Lhermitte-Duclos disease, LDD)
- Associated Abnormalities
  - Meningioma, vascular malformation
  - Predisposition to breast, thyroid, and uterine cancers
  - Autism
- Genetics and Etiology
  - Mutations in the PTEN, tumor suppressor gene
  - Autosomal dominant inheritance or de novo
- Diagnostic Test
  - Brain MRI to detect asymptomatic LDD, vascular malformation, and meningioma

References

Original:
Lloyd KM, Dennis M. Cowden's disease. A possible new symptom complex with multiple system involvement. Ann Intern Med 1963;58:136–142.
[Named Cowden after the surname of the patient]

Review and Case Reports:
Lok C, Viseux V, Avril MF, et al. Brain magnetic resonance imaging in patients with Cowden syndrome. Medicine (Baltimore) 2005 Mar;84(2):129–136.
Elia M, Amato C, Bottitta M, et al. An atypical patient with Cowden syndrome and PTEN gene mutation presenting with cortical malformation and focal epilepsy. Brain Dev 2012 Nov;34:873–876.

Cranial Nerve Syndromes
(alt: Extramedullary cranial nerve syndromes)

Syndrome	Site	Cranial nerve
Foix	Sphenoidal fissure	III, IV, ophthalmic, V, VI
Tolosa-Hunt	Cavernous sinus	III, IV, ophthalmic, V, VI
Jaccoud	Retrospenoidal fossa	II, III, IV, V, VI
Gradenigo	Petrous bone apex	V, VI
Vernet	Jugular foramen	IX, X, XI
Collet-Sicard	Posterior laterocondylar	IX, X, XI, XII
Villaret	Posterior retroparotid	IX, X, XI, XII, Horner syndrome
Tapia	Posterior retroparotid	X, XI, XII

Modified from Ropper AH, Samuels MA. Eds: Adams and Victor's Principles of Neurology, ninth edition; New York, McGraw Hill, 2009. Also, see individual syndromes

CRASH Syndrome
(alt: MASA syndrome)

- Organs Involved
  - Brain, thumbs

- Diagnostic Characteristics
  - *M*ental retardation
  - *A*phasia
  - *S*huffling gait
  - *A*dducted thumbs

- MASA Reclassified as CRASH
  - *C*orpus callosum hypoplasia
  - *R*etardation
  - *A*dducted thumbs
  - *S*pastic paraplegia
  - *H*ydrocephalus

- Genetics
  - X-linked recessive disorders
  - Both MASA and CRASH due to mutations in the L1CAM gene
  - Males affected; female carriers
  - 50 % risk of transfer of affected X chromosome to sons

References

Original:
Bianchine JW, Lewis RC. The MASA syndrome: a new heritable mental retardation syndrome. Clin Genet 1974;5(4):298–306.

Review and Case Reports:
Fransen E, Lemmon V, Van Camp G, Vits L, Coucke P, Williams PJ. CRASH syndrome: clinical spectrum of corpus callosum hypoplasia, retardation, adducted thumbs, spastic paraparesis and hydrocephalus due to mutations in one single gene, L1. Eur J Hum Genet 1995;3(5):273–284.
Yamasaki M, Thompson P, Lemmon V. CRASH syndrome: mutations in L1CAM correlate with severity of the disease. Neuropediatrics 1997 Jun;28(3):175–178.

Cri du Chat Syndrome
(alt: 5p deletion syndrome)

- Organs Involved
  - Microcephaly
  - Hypertelorism, downslanting palpebral fissures, strabismus
  - Micrognathia, low-set ears
  - Single palmar creases, short fingers
  - Cardiac defects
  - Intellectual disability, speech and motor delay
  - Coarsening of facial features in adolescence
  - Small testes

- Associated Abnormalities
  - Cleft lip and palate, excessive drooling
  - Megacolon, horseshoe kidneys
  - Talipes equinovarus, syndactyly
  - Behavior problems, hyperactivity, tantrums

- Genetics
  - Partial deletion of short arm of chromosome 5, 90 % de novo, paternal.
  - Band 5p15.3 is the critical region for catlike cry.
  - Genes involved are SEMAF, CTNND2, and hTERT.

References

Original:
Lejeune J., Lafourcade J, Berger R, et al. Three cases of partial deletion of the short arm of chromosome 5. CR Hebd Seances Acad Sci 1963;257:3098–3102.

Review and Case Reports:
Cerruti Mainardi P. Cri du Chat syndrome. Orphanet J Rare Dis 2006 Sep 5;1:33.

Crouzon Syndrome
(alt: Craniofacial dysostosis)

- Organs Involved
  - First branchial (or pharyngeal) arch, precursor of maxilla and mandible, skull, and sutures
- Diagnostic Characteristics
  - Cranial synostosis, brachycephaly, oxycephaly
  - Exophthalmos, hypertelorism, beak-like nose
  - External strabismus, hearing loss
  - Hypoplastic maxilla, mandibular prognathism
  - Defect of white matter formation
- Associated Abnormalities
  - Brain malformations: Chiari 1, ventriculomegaly, agenesis of corpus callosum, agenesis of septum pellucidum, temporal white matter loss
  - Congenital heart malformations: patent ductus, aortic coarctation
- Genetics
  - Mutation in FGFR2 and 3 (fibroblast growth factor receptors) located on chromosome 10

References

Original:
Crouzon LEO. Dysostose cranio-faciale hereditaire. Bulletin de la Societe des Medecins des Hopitaux de Paris. 1912;33:545–555.

Review and Case Reports:
Raybaud C, Di Rocco C. Brain malformation in syndromic craniosynostosis, a primary disorder of white matter: a review. Childs Nerv Syst 2007 Dec;23(12):1379–1388.

D

Dandy Walker Syndrome – Duane Syndrome

Dandy Walker Syndrome
Deafness-Dystonia-Optic Neuronopathy Syndrome
Dejerine-Roussy Syndrome
Dejerine Syndromes
De Morsier Syndrome
DiGeorge Syndrome
Donnai-Barrow Syndrome
Doose Syndrome
Dravet Syndrome
Duane Syndrome

J.G. Millichap, *Neurological Syndromes: A Clinical Guide to Symptoms and Diagnosis*, DOI 10.1007/978-1-4614-7786-0_4,
© Springer Science+Business Media New York 2013

Dandy Walker Syndrome

- Organs Involved
  - Posterior fossa, cerebellum, 4th ventricle
- Diagnostic Characteristics
  - Agenesis of cerebellar vermis
  - Atresia of foramina of Luschka and Magendie
  - Enlarged posterior fossa
  - Cystic 4th ventricle
  - Elevated tentorium
- Associated Abnormalities
  - Hydrocephalus
  - Increased intracranial pressure
  - Absence of corpus callosum
  - Malformations of heart, face, and limbs
  - Spina bifida
- Differential Diagnosis
  - Dandy Walker syndrome variant, milder form
- Genetics
  - Sporadic ciliopathy
  - Deletion of genes ZIC1 and ZIC4
- Treatment
  - Shunt procedure or 3rd ventriculostomy
  - Rehabilitation therapies
  - Genetic counseling

References

Original:

Benda CE. The Dandy-Walker syndrome or the so-called atresia of the foramen of Magendie. Jrnl Neuropath and Exper Neurol 1954;13:14–39.

Dandy WE, Blackfan KD. Internal hydrocephalus: an experimental, clinical and pathological study. Am J Dis Children, Chicago 1914;8:406–482. Idem 1917;14:424–443.

Walker AEA. A case of congenital atresia of the foramina of Luschka and Magendie: Surgical cure. Jrnl Neuropath and Exper Neurol 1944;3:368–373.

Review and Case Report:

Grinberg I, Northrup H, Ardinger H, Prasad C, Dobyns WB, Millen KJ. Heterozygous deletion of the linked genes ZIC1 and ZIC4 is involved in Dandy-Walker malformation. Nat Genet 2004 Oct;36(10):1053–1055.

Blank MC, Grinberg I, Aryee E, et al. Multiple developmental programs are altered by loss of Zic1 and Zic4 to cause Dandy-Walker malformation cerebellar pathogenesis. Development 2011 Mar;138(6):1207–1216.

Deafness-Dystonia-Optic Neuronopathy Syndrome
(alt: Mohr-Tranebjaerg syndrome)

- Organs Involved
  - Inner ear, brain, eye
- Diagnostic Characteristics
  - Sensorineural hearing loss, profound by age 10 years
  - Dystonia, ataxia
  - Cortical visual impairment, blind in mid-adulthood
  - Changes in personality and aggressive or paranoid behavior
  - Dementia by 40 year of age
- Genetics
  - Mutations in the TIMM8A gene that affect function of mitochondria
  - X-linked recessive progressive disorder

References

Original:
Mohr J, Mageroy K. Sex-linked deafness of a possibly new type. Acta Genet Stat Med 1960;10:54–62.

Review and Case Reports:
Ha AD, Parratt KL, Rendtorff ND, et al. The phenotypic spectrum of dystonia in Mohr-Tranebjaerg syndrome. Mov Disord 2012 Jul;27(8):1034–1040.
Binder J, Hofmann S, Kreisel S, et al. Clinical and molecular findings in a patient with a novel mutation in the deafness-dystonia peptide (DDP1) gene. Brain 2003 Aug;126(Pt 8):1814–1820.

Dejerine-Roussy Syndrome
(alt: Thalamic pain syndrome; central poststroke pain syndrome)

- ■ Organs Involved
  - • Thalamus
- ■ Diagnostic Characteristics
  - • Numbness, burning, and tingling following a thalamic stroke
  - • Severe and chronic pain (dysesthesia or allodynia), not proportional to the touch or pressure stimulus, developing weeks to months later in the hemiplegic side
- ■ Differential Diagnosis
  - • MS
  - • Spinal cord injury
  - • Syringomyelia
  - • Vascular malformation
- ■ Treatment
  - • Tricyclic antidepressants
  - • Anticonvulsant gabapentin
  - • Neurostimulation
- ■ Prognosis
  - • Often refractory and persistent

References

Original:
Dejerine J, Roussy G. Le syndrome thalamique. Rev Neurol (Paris) 1906;14:521–532.

Review and Case Reports:
Klit H, Finnerup NB, Jensen TS. Central post-stroke pain: clinical characteristics, pathophysiology, and management. The Lancet Neurology 2009 Sep;8(9):857–868.

Dejerine Syndromes

Eponym	Syndrome
Dejerine cortical sensory syndrome	Loss of proprioception and stereognosis due to parietal lobe lesion; retained touch, pain, and temperature
Dejerine onion-peel sensory loss	Loss of sensation starting at mouth and nose and spreading outward concentrically, due to lesion in V-trigeminal nucleus
Dejerine medial medullary syndrome	Hypoglossal alternating hemiplegia, anterior spinal artery occlusion, tongue deviates to ipsilateral side, contralateral hemiplegia and hemisensory loss of touch, proprioception, and vibration sense
Dejerine-Klumpke paralysis	Birth injury to lower brachial plexus, weakness of hand muscles, ulnar sensory loss, Horner syndrome
Dejerine-Mouzon syndrome	Impaired primary sensation (pain, thermal, tactile, vibratory) due to parietal lobe lesion
Dejerine-Roussy thalamic syndrome	Hemisensory loss due to thalamic lesion, usually vascular or tumor, position sense most frequently; unpleasant thalamic pain with recovery
Dejerine-Sottas disease	Hypertrophic neuropathy of infancy (CMT3 or HMSN III)
Dejerine-Thomas syndrome	Olivopontocerebellar atrophy, chronic progressive ataxia
Landouzy-Dejerine dystrophy	Facioscapulohumeral muscular dystrophy, autosomal dominant inheritance

Derived from Ropper AH, Samuels MA. Eds. Adams and Vistor's Principles of Neurology, ninth edition; New York, McGraw Hill, 2009. Also, see individual syndromes

D Dandy Walker Syndrome – Duane Syndrome

De Morsier Syndrome
(alt: Septo-optic dysplasia)

- ■ Organs Involved
  - Optic nerves, pituitary gland, septum pellucidum

- ■ Diagnostic Characteristics
  - Optic nerve hypoplasia
  - Absent septum pellucidum
  - Hypopituitarism, growth hormone deficiency

- ■ Associated Abnormalities
  - Congenital nystagmus, small optic disc, hyperplastic vitreous
  - Variable visual impairment
  - Digital defects
  - Hyperbilirubinemia
  - Seizures
  - In utero drug exposure (cocaine, valproate, recreational)
  - Heterotopias, arachnoid cysts

- ■ Genetics
  - Sporadic birth defect of unknown cause.
  - HESX1 mutations are uncommon cause.

- ■ Treatment
  - Hormone replacement therapy

References

Original:
de Morsier G. Etudes sur les dysgraphies, cranioencephaliques III. Agenesie du septum palludi-cum avec malformation du tractus optique. La dysplasie septo-optique. Schweizer Archiv fur Neurologie und Psychiatrie, Zurich 1956;77:267–292.

Review and Case Report:
Webb EA, Dattani MT. Septo-optic dysplasia. Eur J Hum Genet 2010 Apr;18(4):393–397.
Tas E, Tracy M, Sarco DP, Eksioglu YZ, Prabhu SP, Loddenkemper T. Septo-optic dysplasia com-plicated by infantile spasms and bilateral choroidal fissure arachnoid cysts. J Neuroimaging 2011 Jan;21(1):89–91.

DiGeorge Syndrome
(alt: 22q11.2 deletion syndrome, velocardiofacial syndrome, Shprintzen syndrome, conotruncal anomaly face syndrome, Strong syndrome, congenital thymic aplasia)

- Organs Involved
  - Palate, heart, face, nervous system, renal, parathyroid

- Diagnostic Characteristics of CATCH-22
  - C: Cardiac abnormality (tetralogy of Fallot)
  - A: Abnormal facies (hypertelorism)
  - T: Thymic aplasia
  - C: Cleft palate
  - H: Hypocalcemia/hypoparathyroidism
  - 22-Chromosome abnormality

- Associated Abnormalities
  - Learning and expressive language deficits (90 %)
  - Speech hypernasality, delayed vocabulary acquisition, and dysarthria
  - Specific neuropsychological profile, borderline IQ
  - Schizophrenia
  - Seizures (with or without hypocalcemia)
  - Hearing loss (conductive and sensorineural)
  - Basal ganglia and periventricular calcification
  - Autoimmune disorders

- Genetics
  - De novo deletions on chromosome 22q11.2
  - One in two chance of passing deletion 22q to offspring
  - Autosomal recessive or X-linked traits

- Treatment
  - Identify immune problems and treat early
  - Cardiac surgery often required
  - Vitamin D and calcium for hypoparathyroidism
  - Neuropsychological testing and IEP (individual education program)

References

Original:
DiGeorge AM. Congenital absence of the thymus and its immunologic consequences: concurrence with congenital hypoparathyroidism. White Plains, NY: March of Dimes-Birth Defects Foundation. 1968;IV(1):116–121.

D Dandy Walker Syndrome – Duane Syndrome

Review and Case Report:

Kinoshita H, Kokudo T, Ide T, et al. A patient with DiGeorge syndrome with spina bifida and sacral myelomeningocele who developed both hypocalcemia-induced seizure and epilepsy. Seizure 2010 Jun;19(5):303–305.

Robin NH, Shprintzen RJ. Defining the clinical spectrum of deletion 22q11.2. J Pediatr 2005;147(1):90–96.

D   Dandy Walker Syndrome – Duane Syndrome

Donnai-Barrow Syndrome
(alt: Faciooculoacousticorenal (FOAR) syndrome)

- Organs Involved
  - Face, eyes, inner ear, corpus callosum, diaphragm

- Diagnostic Characteristics
  - Agenesis of corpus callosum
  - Large anterior fontanelle
  - Myopia, iris coloboma
  - Hypertelorism, downslanting eyes
  - Severe sensorineural deafness
  - Congenital diaphragmatic hernia

- Genetics
  - Autosomal recessive with mutations in the LRP2 gene on chromosome 2
  - Uniparental disomy reported in some cases, reducing risk of recurrence in a family

References

Original:

Donnai D, Barrow M. Diaphragmatic hernia, exomphalos, absent corpus callosum, hypertelorism, myopia, and sensorineural deafness: A newly recognized autosomal recessive disorder? Am J Med Genet 1993;47:679–682.

Review and Case Report:

Kantarci S, Ragge NK, Thomas NS, et al. Donnai-Barrow syndrome (DBS/FOAR) in a child with a homozygous LRP2 mutation due to complete chromosome 2 paternal isodisomy. Am J Med Genet Part A 2008;146A:1842–1847.

Doose Syndrome
(alt: Myoclonic-astatic epilepsy)

- ■ Diagnostic Characteristics
  - Onset between 7 months and 6 years of age.
  - Normal development before onset.
  - Ratio of boys to girls 2:1.
  - Myoclonic-astatic seizures (sudden falls, head nodding without loss of consciousness) define syndrome.
  - Absence with atonic and generalized tonic-clonic seizures also occurs.
  - Status epilepticus and nonconvulsive status are common.
  - Interictal EEG generalized 2–3 Hz spikes-/polyspike-and-waves.
  - Ictal EEG spike or polyspike waves at 2.5–3 Hz.

- ■ Differential Diagnosis
  - Benign or progressive myoclonic epilepsies
  - Dravet syndrome
  - Lennox-Gastaut syndrome

- ■ Genetics
  - Multifactorial inheritance likely. Specific gene not identified
  - High familial incidence of epilepsy

- ■ Treatment
  - Valproate, levetiracetam, and clobazam are effective in idiopathic cases.
  - Carbamazepine, phenytoin, and vigabatrin worsen MAS.
  - Ketogenic diet is probably the most effective treatment.

- ■ Prognosis
  - Variable. Good in idiopathic cases, with normal neurodevelopment (80 %)
  - Poor outcome with status

References

Original:
Doose H, Gerken H, Leonhardt R, Volzke E, Volz C. Centrencephalic myoclonic-astatic petit mal. Clinical and genetic investigations. Neuropediatrie 1970;2:59–78.

Review and Case Reports:
Ebach K, Joos H, Doose H, et al. SCN1A mutation analysis in myoclonic astatic epilepsy and sever idiopathic generalized epilepsy of infancy with generalized tonic-clonic seizures. Neuropediatrics 2005 Jun;36(3):210–213.
Kelley SA, Kossoff EH. Doose syndrome (myoclonic-astatic epilepsy): 40 years of progress. Dev Med Child Neurol 2010 Nov;52(11):988–993.

Dravet Syndrome
(alt: Severe myoclonic epilepsy of infancy (SMEI))

- Diagnostic Characteristics
  - Onset with febrile seizure in the first year of life. Early development is normal.
  - Myoclonic seizures begin between 1 and 4 years of age.
  - Convulsive status epilepticus and alternating hemiconvulsions are common.
  - EEG normal at onset; generalized spike-and-wave or polyspike-and-wave.
  - Psychomotor development is delayed from second year of life.
  - Seizures are often resistant to medication.
  - Ataxia.
  - "Borderline" cases of DS (SMEB) have SMEI with less frequent seizures.

- Differential Diagnosis
  - Febrile seizures or febrile status epilepticus
  - Severe infantile multifocal epilepsy (SIMFE)
  - Benign myoclonic epilepsy (BME)
  - Lennox-Gastaut syndrome
  - Myoclonic-astatic epilepsy (MAE) (Doose syndrome)

- Genetics
  - >70 % cases have mutations of SCN1A gene, most de novo.
  - Family history of epilepsy or febrile seizures in ~25 % cases.

- Treatment
  - Avoid carbamazepine and lamotrigine, AEDs that exacerbate SMEI.
  - Valproate, topiramate, clobazam, and levetiracetam are partially effective.
  - Ketogenic diet is an alternative or supplement to AEDs.
  - Avoid triggers such as hot baths.

- Prognosis
  - Seizures are usually only partially controlled and may persist through adult life.

References

Original:
Dravet C, Roger J, Bureau M, Dalla Bernardina M. Myoclonic epilepsies in childhood. In: Akimoto H. Kazamatsuri H, Seino M, Ward A, eds. Advances in Epileptology: XIIIth Epilepsy International Symposium. New York: Raven Press; 1982:135–141.

Engel J Jr. A proposed diagnostic scheme for people with epileptic seizures and with epilepsy: report of the ILAE Task Force on Classification and Terminology. Epilepsia 2001;42:796–803.

Reviews and Case Reports:

Korff C, Laux L, Kelley K, Goldstein J, Koh S, Nordli DR Jr. Dravet syndrome (severe myoclonic epilepsy in infancy): a retrospective study of 16 patients. J Child Neurol 2007;22:185–194.

Millichap JJ, Koh S, Laux LC, Nordli DR Jr. Child Neurology: Dravet syndrome. When to suspect the diagnosis. Neurology 2009 Sep 29;73(13):e59–62.

Dravet C. The core Dravet syndrome phenotype. Epilepsia 2011 Apr;52 Suppl 2:3–9.

D Dandy Walker Syndrome – Duane Syndrome

Duane Syndrome
(alt: Stilling-Turk-Duane syndrome)

- Organs Involved
  - Eye, sixth cranial nerve and nucleus, lateral rectus muscle

- Diagnostic Characteristics
  - Limitation of abduction of affected eye.
  - Retraction of eyeball on adduction and narrowing of palpebral fissure.
  - Limited convergence.
  - Face turned to affected side to maintain binocular vision.
  - When unaffected right eye looks to right, affected left eye looks straight.

- Associated Abnormalities (Duane's Plus)
  - Cervical spine abnormalities (Klippel-Feil syndrome)
  - Goldenhar syndrome
  - Heterochromia

- Epidemiology
  - Girls affected > boys, 3:2
  - 10–20 % familial

- Classification
  - Two systems of classification: Brown's A, B, and C; Huber's types I, II, and III

- Differential Diagnosis
  - Acquired causes, trauma, orbital infection
  - VI cranial nerve palsy

- Treatment
  - None required in most cases
  - Surgery when patient unable to maintain binocular vision

References

Original:
Duane A. Congenital deficiency of abduction associated with impairment of adduction, retraction movements, contraction of the palpebral fissure and oblique movements of the eye. Arch Ophthalmol (Chicago) 1905;34:133–150.

Reviews and Case Reports:
Mohan K, Sharma A, Panday SS. Differences in epidemiological and clinical characteristics between various types of Duane retraction syndrome in 331 patients. JAAPOS 2008 Dec;12(6): 576–580.
Alexandrakis G, Saunders RA. Duane retraction syndrome. Ophthalmol Clin North Am 2001 Sep;14(3):407–417.

E

Edwards Syndrome – Epilepsy (Electroclinical) Syndromes

Edwards Syndrome
Elsberg Syndrome
Empty Sella Syndrome (ESS)
Epidermal Nevus Syndrome
Epilepsy (Electroclinical) Syndromes

J.G. Millichap, *Neurological Syndromes: A Clinical Guide to Symptoms and Diagnosis*, DOI 10.1007/978-1-4614-7786-0_5,
© Springer Science+Business Media New York 2013

Edwards Syndrome
(alt: Trisomy 18 syndrome)

- Organs Involved
  - Kidneys, heart, intestine, brain, muscle, extremities
- Diagnostic Characteristics
  - Kidney malformation
  - Ventricular septal defect
  - Omphalocele, esophageal atresia
  - Mental retardation
  - Growth deficiency
  - Arthrogryposis
- Associated Abnormalities
  - Microcephaly, prominent occiput, choroid plexus cysts
  - Low-set, malformed ears; upturned nose
  - Micrognathia, cleft lip/palate
  - Hypertelorism, ptosis, narrow palpebral fissures
  - Clenched hands, underdeveloped thumbs or nails, webbed 2nd and 3rd toes
  - Absent radius, clubfoot or Rocker bottom feet
  - Undescended testicles
- Genetics
  - Extra copy of genetic material on chromosome 18
  - Trisomy 18 (47, XX, +18)
  - More prevalent in female offspring
- Prognosis
  - 50 % of infants do not survive beyond first week of life
  - Median life span 5–15 days, 8 % >1 year, 1 % to age 10 year (mosaic cases)

References

Original:
Edwards JH, Harnden DG, Cameron AH, Crosse VM, Wolff OH. A new trisomic syndrome. The Lancet 1960;1:787–790.

Review and Case Reports:
Boghosian-Sell L, Mewar R, Harrison W, et al. Molecular mapping of the Edwards syndrome phenotype to two noncontiguous regions on chromosome 18. Am J Hum Genet 1994 Sep;55(3):476–483.
Moyano D, Huggon IC, Allan LD. Fetal echocardiography in trisomy 18. Arch Dis Child Fetal Neonatal Ed 2005 Nov;90(6):F520–522.

Elsberg Syndrome

- ▪ Organs Involved
  - • Bladder, vulva, cauda equina

- ▪ Diagnostic Characteristics
  - • Acute urinary retention
  - • Herpes genitalis infection
  - • Viral radiculomyelitis
  - • CSF lymphocytosis

- ▪ Differential Diagnosis
  - • Tumor of cauda equina
  - • Multiple sclerosis

References

Original:
Elsberg CA. Experiences in spinal surgery. Observation upon 60 laminectomies for spinal disease. Surg Gynecol Obstet 1931;16:117–135.

Review and Case Report:
Caplan LR, Kleeman FJ, Berg S. Urinary retension probably secondary to herpes genitalis. N Engl J Med 1977;297:920–921.
Vanneste JA, Karthaus PP, Davies G. Acute urinary retention due to sacral myeloradiculitis. J Neurol Neurosurg Psychiatry 1980;43:954–956.
Lepori P, Marcacci G, Gaglianone S. Elsberg syndrome: radiculomyelopathy and acute urinary retention in patient with genital herpes. Italian J Neurological Sci 1992 May;13(4):373–375.

Empty Sella Syndrome (ESS)

- ■ Organs Involved
  - Sella turcica, pituitary gland, hypothalamus
- ■ Diagnostic Characteristics
  - Primary ESS: sign of idiopathic intracranial hypertension, commonly with obesity and high blood pressure in women; defect in the dural diaphragm with herniation of third ventricle into empty sella
  - Secondary ESS: pituitary gland atrophy due to injury, surgery, or radiation therapy
- ■ Associated Abnormalities
  - Early onset of puberty, growth hormone deficiency, pituitary dysfunction
  - Pituitary tumor
  - Hypothalamic hypopituitarism
  - Hyperprolactinemia
- ■ Diagnosis
  - MRI and endocrine evaluation

References

Thwin M, Brophy BP. Hyperprolactinemia and the empty sella. J Clin Neurosci 2012 Apr;19(4):605–606.

Komada H, Yamamoto M, Okubo S, et al. A case of hypothalamic panhypopituitarism with empty sella syndrome: case report and review of the literature. Endocr J 2009;56(4):585–589.

Nishi Y, Hamamoto K, Fujita N, Okada S. Empty sella/pituitary atrophy and endocrine impairments as a consequence of radiation and chemotherapy in long-term survivors of childhood leukemia. Int J Hematol 2011 Oct;94(4):399–402.

Kaufman B, Tomsak RL, Kaufman RA, et al. Herniation of the suprasellar visual system and third ventricle into empty sella. Morphologic and clinical considerations. AJR Am J Roentgenol. 1989;152:597.

Epidermal Nevus Syndrome
(alt: Solomon's syndrome)

- Organs Involved
  - Skin, central nervous system, skeleton

- Diagnostic Characteristics
  - Epidermal nevi, various (ichthyosis, acanthotic, sebaceous)
  - Neurological abnormalities in 50 %: mental retardation 40 %, epilepsy 30 %
  - Ocular abnormalities in 33 %, coloboma, microphthalmia, cataracts
  - Skeletal, cardiac, and urogenital abnormalities

- Associated Abnormalities
  - Ipsilateral hemihypertrophy
  - Hemimegalencephaly
  - Seizures, focal, infantile spasms, EEG abnormal side of nevus
  - Developmental delay, sensorineural deafness
  - Spastic hemiparesis, cortical atrophy, ventricle enlargement
  - Kyphoscoliosis, hip dislocation, polydactyly
  - Brainstem and cerebellar malformations; neonatal medulloblastoma

- Differential Diagnosis
  - Proteus syndrome
  - CHILD syndrome
  - Becker nevus syndrome with ipsilateral breast hypoplasia

- Genetics
  - Sporadic, congenital acquired, not hereditary

- Treatment
  - Surgery, abrasion. Control of seizures

- Prognosis
  - Rare tendency to malignant transformation, especially nevus sebaceous
  - Rare associated visceral malignancies (Wilm's tumor, astrocytoma, intrathoracic teratoma, etc.). Nevi often amenable to therapy

References

Original:
Solomon LM, Fretzin DF, Dewald RL. The epidermal nevus syndrome. Arch Dermatol 1968;97: 273–285.

Review and Case Reports:
Egan CA, Meadows KP, Van Orman CB, Vanderhooft SL. Neurologic variant of epidermal nevus syndrome with a facial lipoma. Int J Dermatol 2001;40:189–190.
Brandling-Bennett HA, Morel KD. Epidermal nevi. Pediatr Clin North Am 2010 Oct;57(5): 1177–1198.
Okumura A, Lee T, Ikeno M, et al. Case report. Brain Dev 2012 Nov;34:881–885.

E Edwards Syndrome – Epilepsy (Electroclinical) Syndromes

Epilepsy (Electroclinical) Syndromes

(Table modified from Berg AT et al. Revised terminology and concepts for organization of seizures and epilepsies: Report of the ILAE Commission on Classification and Terminology, 2005–2009. Epilepsia 2010;51(4):676–685)

- Listed by Age at Onset
  - *Neonatal*
  - Benign familial neonatal epilepsy
  - Early myoclonic encephalopathy
  - Ohtahara syndrome
  - *Infancy*
  - West syndrome
  - Myoclonic epilepsy in infancy
  - Benign infantile epilepsy
  - Dravet syndrome
  - *Childhood*
  - Febrile seizures plus (FS+)
  - Panayiotopoulos syndrome
  - Myoclonic-atonic (astatic) seizures
  - Benign epilepsy with centrotemporal spikes (BECTS)
  - Autosomal-dominant nocturnal frontal lobe epilepsy (ADNFLE)
  - Late-onset childhood occipital epilepsy (Gastaut type)
  - Lennox-Gastaut syndrome
  - Epileptic encephalopathy with continuous spike-and-wave during sleep (CSWS)
  - Landau-Kleffner syndrome (LKS)
  - Childhood absence epilepsy (CAE)
  - *Adolescence–Adult*
  - Juvenile absence epilepsy (JAE)
  - Juvenile myoclonic epilepsy (JME) (Janz syndrome)
  - Epilepsy with generalized tonic-clonic seizures alone
  - Progressive myoclonus epilepsies (PME)
  - Autosomal-dominant epilepsy with auditory features (ADEAF)
  - Other familial temporal lobe epilepsies
  - Reflex epilepsies

- Distinctive Constellations
  - Mesial temporal lobe epilepsy with hippocampal sclerosis (MTLE with HS)
  - Rasmussen syndrome
  - Gelastic seizures with hypothalamic hamartoma
  - Hemiconvulsion-hemiplegia epilepsy

- Structural-Metabolic Etiologies
  - Malformations of cortical development (heterotopias, agyria, polymicrogyria etc.)
  - Neurocutaneous syndromes (tuberous sclerosis complex, Sturge-Weber syndrome, etc.)
  - Tumor
  - Infection
  - Trauma
  - Vascular

- Epilepsies of Unknown Cause

- Seizures not recognized as an epilepsy: febrile seizures, benign neonatal seizures

E Edwards Syndrome – Epilepsy (Electroclinical) Syndromes

F

Fazio-Londe Syndrome – Froin Syndrome

Fazio-Londe Syndrome
Feingold Syndrome
Ferguson-Critchley Syndrome
Fetal Alcohol Syndrome
Foix-Alajouanine Syndrome
Foix-Chavany-Marie Syndrome
Foster-Kennedy Syndrome
Foville Syndrome
Fragile X Syndrome
Fragile X-Associated Tremor/Ataxia Syndrome
Froehlich Syndrome
Froin Syndrome

J.G. Millichap, *Neurological Syndromes: A Clinical Guide to Symptoms and Diagnosis*, DOI 10.1007/978-1-4614-7786-0_6,
© Springer Science+Business Media New York 2013

Fazio-Londe Syndrome
(alt: Progressive bulbar paresis of childhood)

- Organs Involved
  - Facial, lingual, pharyngeal, laryngeal, and ocular muscles
- Diagnostic Characteristics
  - Onset variable age, usually early childhood, death in first decade
  - Progressive facial diplegia
  - Bulbar paralysis (dysarthria, dysphagia, dysphonia)
  - Tongue fasciculations
- Associated Abnormalities
  - Stridor and respiratory symptoms at onset
  - Oculomotor paresis and jaw weakness in some
  - Loss of motor neurons in hypoglossal, vagus, facial, and trigeminal nuclei
  - Atrophy of pyramidal tracts
- Differential Diagnosis
  - Myasthenia gravis
  - Pontomedullary glioma
  - Brainstem multiple sclerosis
- Genetics
  - Autosomal recessive, either with early onset of respiratory symptoms and rapid progression to death (type I) or less prominent respiratory symptoms and protracted clinical course (type II)
  - Rare autosomal dominant form (type III) and very rarely X-linked form

References

Original:
Fazio M. Ereditarieta della paralisi bulbare progressive. Reforma Medica1892;8:327.
Londe P. Paralysie bulbaire progressive infantile et familiale. Rev Med 1894;14:212–254.

Reviews and Case Reports:
Gomez MR, Clermont V, Bernstein J. Progressive bulbar paralysis in childhood (Fazio-Londe's disease). Arch Neurol, Chicago. 1962;6:317–323.
McShane MA, Boyd S, Harding B, Brett EM, Wilson J. Progressive bulbar paralysis of childhood. A reappraisal of Fazio-Londe disease. Brain 1992 Dec;115(Pt 6):1889–1900.
Markand ON, Daly DD. Juvenile type of slowly progressive bulbar palsy. Report of a case. Neurology 1971;21:753.

Feingold Syndrome
(alt: Oculodigitoesophagoduodenal syndrome)

- Organs Involved
  - Head, limbs, intestines, brain, eyes

- Diagnostic Characteristics
  - Microcephaly
  - Clinodactyly, short index and little fingers
  - Syndactyly of 2nd and 3rd and 4th and 5th toe
  - Short palpebral fissures
  - Esophageal and/or duodenal atresia
  - Learning disability or mental retardation

- Genetics
  - Mutations in the neuroblastoma-derived oncogene (MYCN), located on the short arm of chromosome 2 (2p24.1)

References

Original:

Feingold M. Case report 30. Syndrome Identification 1975;3(1):16–17.

Feingold M. An unusual microcephaly. Hospital Practice 1978;13:44–49.

Review and Case Report:

Dodds A, Ramsden R, Kingston H. Feingold syndrome – a cause of profound deafness. J Laryngol & Otol 1999 Oct;113(10):919–921.

Courtens W, Levi S, Verbelen F, Verloes A, Varnos E. Feingold syndrome: report of a new family and review. Am J Med Genet 1997 Nov 28;73(1):55–60.

Ferguson-Critchley Syndrome

- ■ Organs Involved
  - Eyes, spinocerebellar, brain
- ■ Diagnostic Characteristics
  - Cerebellar ataxia of late onset, fourth and fifth decades
  - Spastic paraparesis
  - Supranuclear ophthalmoplegia, optic atrophy
  - Myoclonus
  - Dementia
- ■ Associated Abnormalities
  - Pathologic crying and laughing
  - Dysarthria
  - Sensation diminished distally
  - Extrapyramidal features in some families
- ■ Genetics
  - Autosomal dominant inheritance, several families reported
  - Mutations in the SCA3 gene
  - Drew family of Walworth described by Ferguson and Critchley in 1929

References

Original:
Ferguson FR, Critchley M. A clinical study of an heredo-familial disease resembling disseminated sclerosis. Brain 1929;52:20–225.

Review and Case Reports:
Harding AE. The clinical features and classification of the late onset autosomal dominant cerebellar ataxias. A study of 11 families, including descendants of the 'the Drew family of Walworth'. Brain 1982 Mar;105(Pt 1):1–28.
Teive HA, Arruda WO. The Drew family of Walworth: one century from the first evaluation until the final diagnosis, Machado-Joseph disease. Arq Neuropsiquiatr 2004 Mar;62(1):177–180.

Fetal Alcohol Syndrome

- ■ Organs Involved
  - • Face, brain, eyes, heart, skeleton, kidneys
- ■ Diagnostic Characteristics
  - • Growth deficiency
  - • Craniofacial abnormalities: smooth philtrum, thin upper lip, small palpebral fissures
  - • CNS damage: microcephaly, agenesis of corpus callosum, cerebellar hypoplasia; epilepsy, incoordination, cognitive and behavioral abnormalities (developmental delay, learning disabilities, ADHD)
  - • Prenatal exposure to alcohol
- ■ Associated Abnormalities
  - • Strabismus, ptosis,
  - • Cardiac ventricular and atrial septal defects
  - • Joint anomalies, single palmar crease, small phalanges and nails
- ■ Differential Diagnosis
  - • Williams syndrome
  - • Noonan syndrome
  - • Fetal hydantoin syndrome

References

Original:
Sullivan WC. A note on the influence of maternal inebriety on the offspring. Jrnl Mental Science 1899;45:489–503.
Jones KL, Smith DW, Ulleland CN, Streissguth AP. Pattern of malformation in offspring of chronic alcoholic mothers. Lancet 1973;1:1267–1271.

Review and Case Reports:
Bell SH, Stade B, Reynolds JN, et al. The remarkably high prevalence of epilepsy and seizure history in fetal alcohol spectrum disorders. Alcohol Clin Exp Res 2010 Jun;34(6):1084–1089.
Riley EP, Infante MA, Warren KR. Fetal alcohol spectrum disorders: an overview. Neuropsychol Rev 2011 Jun;21(2):73–80.

Foix-Alajouanine Syndrome
(alt: Foix-Alajouanine myelopathy; subacute necrotic myelopathy)

- ■ Organs Involved
  - • Spinal cord, spinal blood vessels
- ■ Diagnostic Characteristics
  - • Progressive spastic paraplegia
  - • Flaccid areflexive paraplegia
  - • Sensory loss, loss of sphincter control
  - • CSF protein elevated to >100 mg/dl and no cells
  - • Small tortuous spinal arteries and veins thickened and fibrotic (angio-dysplastic) or spinal arteriovenous malformation with vascular myelopathy
  - • Lower thoracic and/or lumbosacral cord, rarely cervical cord
  - • Male: female ratio/5:1
  - • Most common in 20–40-year-olds; fatal within 1–2 years

References

Original:
Foix C, Alajouanine T. Le myelite necrotique subaigue (myelite centrale angiohypertrophique a evolution progressive). Paraplegie amyotrophique lentement ascendante d'abord spasmodique, puis flasque. Revue Neurologique, Paris 1926;2:1–42.

Review and Case Report:
Greenfield JG, Turner JWA. Acute and subacute necrotic myelitis. Brain 1939;62:227.
Ropper AH, Samuels MA. Eds Adams and Victor's Principles of Neurology, ninth edition, New York, McGraw Hill, 2009.

Foix-Chavany-Marie Syndrome

- ■ Organs Involved
  - • Face, pharynx, tongue, masticatory muscles, opercular cortex, cerebral arteries
- ■ Diagnostic Characteristics
  - • Facial apraxic weakness
  - • Anarthria, drooling
  - • Dysphagia, masticatory problems
  - • Exaggerated jaw jerk
  - • Closes mouth spontaneously when smiling but not voluntarily
- ■ Causes
  - • Stroke affecting the cerebral anterior opercular region, usually bilateral
  - • Cerebral malformation
  - • Degenerative disorder
  - • Head trauma

References

Original:
Foix C, Chavany JA, Marie J. Diplegie facio-linguo-masticatrice d'origine sous-corticale sans paralysie des membres (contribution a l'etude de la localisation des centres de la face du member superieur). Revue Neurologique, Paris 1926;33:214–219.

Review and Case Report:
Ohtomo R, Iwata A, Tsuji S. Unilateral opercular infarction presenting with Foix-Chavany-Marie syndrome. J Stroke Cerebrovasc Dis 2012 Oct 5 [Epub ahead of print]

Foster-Kennedy Syndrome

- Organs Involved
  - Olfactory groove, sphenoid ridge, frontal lobe of brain
- Diagnostic Characteristics
  - Ipsilateral optic atrophy
  - Contralateral papilledema
  - Ipsilateral central scotoma
  - Ipsilateral anosmia
  - Anterior cranial fossa mass (olfactory groove meningioma)
- Associated Abnormalities
  - Increased intracranial pressure
  - Frontal lobe symptoms
- Differential Diagnosis
  - Pseudo-Foster Kennedy syndrome (ipsilateral optic atrophy and contralateral papilledema without mass) due to unilateral optic nerve hypoplasia.
- Treatment
  - Surgery, ventriculoperitoneal shunt

References

Original:
Kennedy F. Retrobulbar neuritis as an exact diagnostic sign of certain tumors and abscesses in the frontal lobes. Am J Med Sci 1911;142:355–368.

Reviews and Case Reports:
Giombini S, Solero CL, Lasio G, et al. Immediate and late outcome of operation for parasagittal and falx meningiomas: report of 342 cases. Surg Neurol 1984;21:427–435.
Acebes X, Arruga J, Acebes JJ, Majos C, Munoz S, Valero IA. Intracranial meningiomatosis causing Foster Kennedy syndrome by unilateral optic nerve compression and blockage of the superior sagittal sinus. J Neuro-Ophthalmology 2009 June;29(2):140–142.
Bansal S, Dabbs T, Long V. Pseudo-Foster Kennedy syndrome due to unilateral optic nerve hypoplasia: a case report. J Med Case Reports 2008;2:86.

Foville Syndrome
(alt: Dorsolateral pontine syndrome; Raymond-Foville syndrome)

- Organs Involved
  - Tegmentum of pons, cranial nerves VI and VII
  - Corticospinal tracts in basis pontis

- Diagnostic Characteristics
  - Ipsilateral Cr VI palsy (lateral gaze weakness with diplopia)
  - Ipsilateral Cr VII palsy (peripheral facial weakness)
  - Contralateral hemiplegia (sparing the face) (crossed hemiplegia)

- Causes
  - Basilar artery infarct (paramedian and short circumferential branches) or pontine tumor
  - Unilateral lesion of the dorsal pons tegmentum

- Differential Diagnosis
  - Other intramedullary brainstem syndromes (Millard-Gubler, Weber, Claude, Benedikt, Nothnagel, Parinaud, Avellis, Jackson, Wallenberg)

References

Original:
Foville ALF. Note sur une paralysie peu connue de certains muscles de l'oeil, et sa liaison avec quelques points de l'anatomie de la physiologie de la protuberance annulaire. Gazette hebdomadair de medicine et de chirurgie. 1859;6:146.

Review and Case Reports:
Wolf JK. The Classical Brainstem Syndromes. Springfield, IL, Charles C Thomas, 1971, for translation of original reports.
Brogna C, Fiengo L, Ture U. Achille Louis Foville's atlas of brain anatomy and the Defoville syndrome. Neurosurgery 2012 May;70(5):1265–1273.

Fragile X Syndrome
(alt: Martin-Bell syndrome)

- Organs Involved
  - Ears, face, testes, brain
- Diagnostic Characteristics
  - Mental retardation or learning disability.
  - Autism (FXS is the leading genetic cause of autism, accounting for 5 % cases).
  - Large protruding ears, long face.
  - Postpubescent macroorchidism.
  - Hyperextensible finger joints, flat feet, hypotonia.
  - Males are affected more than females. Females have 50 % penetrance.
- Associated Abnormalities
  - Stereotypic movements (e.g., hand flapping)
  - Working and short-term memory deficiencies, visual spatial and math learning disabilities. Verbal abilities relatively spared
  - Social anxiety, excessive shyness, panic attacks, autistic spectrum disorder
  - ADHD in majority of boys and 30 % girls with FXS
  - Seizures in 13–18 %, mainly partial seizures, amenable to medication
- Genetics
  - X-linked autosomal is dominant. Genetic anticipation in future generations.
  - Mutation of the fragile X mental retardation 1 (FMR1) gene on the X chromosome, with increase in CGG trinucleotide repeats on PCR analysis.
  - FXS males have >200 repeats (unaffected individuals have 5–44 repeats).
  - Methylation of FMR1 in chromosome Xq27.3 causes constriction of the X chromosome with "fragile" appearance microscopically.
  - FMRP, at highest concentration in brain and testes, affects dopamine pathways in prefrontal cortex, resulting in ADHD.
- Treatment
  - Stimulants for ADHD. Behavioral therapy and special education

References

Original:
Martin JP, Bell J. A pedigree of mental defect showing sex-linkage. J Neurol Psychiat 1943; 6(3–4):154–157.
Lubs HA. A marker X chromosome. Am J Hum Genet 1969 May;21(3):231–244.

Reviews and Case Reports:
Hagerman RJ, Berry-Kravis E, Kaufmann WE, et al. Advances in the treatment of fragile X syndrome. Pediatrics 2009;123(1):378–390.
Murphy MM. A review of mathematical learning disabilities in children with fragile X syndrome. Dev Disabil Res Rev 2009;15(1):21–27.

Fragile X-Associated Tremor/Ataxia Syndrome

- Organs Involved
  - Middle cerebellar peduncles, cerebral white matter, brain atrophy
- Diagnostic Characteristics
  - Late-adult-onset neurodegenerative disease
  - Intention tremor
  - Cerebellar gait ataxia
  - Cognitive dysfunction (executive function, working memory)
- Associated Abnormalities
  - Parkinsonism.
  - Neuropathic and autonomic dysfunction.
  - Intranuclear inclusions (ubiquitin positive) in neurons and astrocytes are the pathological hallmark, especially affecting the hippocampus.
- Genetics
  - A trinucleotide repeat disorder is the fragile X mental retardation 1 gene, FMR1.
  - Men are most often affected and carriers of premutation expansion (55–200 CGG repeats) of the FMR1 gene. Complex multigenerational inheritance.
  - Siblings of patient are at risk. Patient and family members require genetic counseling.
- Treatment
  - None specific, targeting the pathogenic mechanism of excess FMR1 mRNA
  - Supportive therapy for ataxia and Parkinsonism
- Prognosis
  - Progressive, tremors first with onset at median of ~60 years, followed by ataxia after median of 2 years, and death after 21 years.
  - Life expectancy ranges from 5 to 25 years.

References

Original:
Hagerman RJ, Lechey M, Heinrichs W, et al. Intention tremor, parkinsonism, and generalized brain atrophy in male carriers of Fragile X. Neurology 2001;57:127–130.

Reviews and Case Reports:
Berry-Kravis E, Abrams L, Coffey SM, et al. Fragile X-associated tremor/ataxia syndrome: Clinical features, genetics, and testing guidelines. Mov Disord 2007;22(14):2018–2030.
Amiri K, Hagerman RJ, Hagerman PJ. Fragile X-associated tremor/ataxia. An aging face of the fragile X gene. Arch Neurol 2008 Jan;65(1):19–25.

F Fazio-Londe Syndrome – Froin Syndrome

Froehlich Syndrome
(alt: Adiposogenital dystrophy; Babinski-Frohlich syndrome; hypothalamic infantilism)

- Organs Involved
  - Pituitary, hypothalamus

- Diagnostic Characteristics
  - Feminine obesity, growth retardation
  - Retarded sexual development, altered secondary sex characteristics
  - Gonadal underdevelopment or atrophy, decreased gonadotropin secretion
  - Loss of vision, polyuria, polydipsia
  - Antisocial behavior
  - Apathy, increased appetite
  - Mostly males affected, during puberty

- Associated Abnormalities
  - Pituitary tumor
  - Hypothalamic tumor, suprasellar cyst
  - Craniopharyngioma, adamantinoma, glioma
  - Pituitary adenoma, cholesteatoma, lipoma, meningioma, chordoma

- Differential Diagnosis
  - Prader-Willi syndrome

References

Original:

Babinski JF. Tumeur du corps pituitaire sans acromegalie et avec arret de developpement des organs genitaux. Revue Neurologique, Paris. 1900;8:531–535.

Frohlich A. Ein fall von tumor der hypophysis cerebri ohne akromegalie. Wiener Klinische Rundschau. 1901;15:833–836:906–908.

Review and Case Reports:

Zarate A, Saucedo R. The adiposogenital dystrophy or Frohlich syndrome and the beginning of the concept of neuroendocrinology. Gac Med Mex 2007;143(4):349–350.

Ropper AH, Samuels MA. Eds Adams and Victor's Principles of Neurology, ninth edition; New York, McGraw Hill, 2009.

Froin Syndrome
(alt: Nonne-Froin syndrome)

- Organs Involved
  - Cerebrospinal fluid, spinal subarachnoid space
- Diagnostic Characteristics
  - CSF obtained by lumbar puncture is xanthochromic.
  - CSF protein concentration is elevated.
  - Partial or complete block of spinal canal.

References

Original:

Froin G. Inflammations meningees avec reactions chromatique, fibrineuse et cytologique du liquide cephalo-rachidien. Gazette des Hopitaux, Paris. 1903;76:1005–1006.

Review and Case Reports:

Greenfield JG. Original papers: On Froin's syndrome, and its relation to allied conditions in the cerebrospinal fluid. J Neurol Psychopathol 1921 Aug;2(6):105–141.

Williams B. Cerebrospinal fluid pressure changes in response to coughing. Brain 1976 Jun;99(2):331–346.

G

Ganser Syndrome – Guillain-Barre Syndrome

Ganser Syndrome
Garcin Syndrome
Gerstmann Syndrome
Goldenhar Syndrome
Gorlin Syndrome
Gradenigo Syndrome
Greig Cephalopolysyndactyly Syndrome
Guillain-Barre Syndrome

J.G. Millichap, *Neurological Syndromes: A Clinical Guide to Symptoms and Diagnosis*, DOI 10.1007/978-1-4614-7786-0_7,
© Springer Science+Business Media New York 2013

Ganser Syndrome

- ■ Organs Involved
  - • Frontotemporal-parietal dominant lobes of brain
- ■ Diagnostic Characteristics
  - • Dissociative disorder NOS
  - • Approximate, nonsensical, or wrong answers to simple questions or incorrect way of doing things
  - • Clouding of consciousness, hallucinations
  - • Conversion symptoms, hysterical escape (prison psychosis)
- ■ Associated Abnormalities
  - • Organic causes: head injury or stroke, mostly involving frontal lobes
  - • Alcoholism with Korsakoff psychosis, schizophrenia, depression
  - • Neurosyphilis, dementia, or AIDS
  - • Confusion, stress, echolalia, echopraxia
- ■ Age and Gender
  - • Average age 32 years (range 15–62), also reported in children
  - • Most common in men (75 %) and prisoners
- ■ Treatment
  - • Psychiatric care
  - • Neurological consult to rule out organic disease

References

Original:
Ganser SJM. Uber einen eigenartigen hysterischen Dammerzustand. Archiv fur Psychiatrie und Nervenkrankheiten, Berlin. 1898;30:633–640.

Review and Case Report:
Carney MW, Chary TK, Robotis P, Childs A. Ganser syndrome and its management. Brit Jrnl Psychiat: the journal of mental science. 1987;151(5):697–700.
Cocores JA, Schlesinger LB, Gold MS. A review of the EEG literature on Ganser's syndrome. Internat Jrnl of Psychiatry in Medicine. 1986;16(1):59–65.
Miller P, Bramble D, Buxton N. Case study: Ganser syndrome in children and adolescents. J Am Acad Child Adolesc Psychiatry.1997 Jan;36(1):112–115.
Anupama M, Rao KN, Dhananiaya S. Ganser syndrome and lesion in the temporoparietal region. Indian J Psychiatry 2006 Apr-Jun;48(2):123–125.

Garcin Syndrome
(alt: Guillain-Alajouanine-Garcin syndrome)

- Organs Involved
  - Multiple unilateral cranial nerves, nasopharynx, base of skull
- Diagnostic Characteristics
  - Progressive paralyses of cranial nerves on one side
  - Tumor involving the base of the skull: meningeal carcinomatosis, lymphomatosis, nasopharyngeal carcinoma (Schmincke tumor or lymphoepithelioma)
  - Trauma involving base of skull and cranial nerves outside the brainstem
  - Localized, subacute infection (herpes zoster, Lyme disease, cytomegalovirus)
  - Wegener granulomatosis, sarcoidosis
  - Tumors involving cranial nerves: neurofibromas, schwannomas (acoustic), metastases, meningiomas, chordomas, chondrosarcomas

References

Original:
Garcin R. Le syndrome paralytique unilateral globale des nerfs craniens. These de Paris, 1927.

Review and Case Reports:
Keane JR. Multiple cranial nerve palsies: Analysis of 79 cases. Arch Neurol 1975;62:1714.
Ropper AH, Samuels MA. Eds Adams and Victor's Principles of Neurology, ninth edition, New York, McGraw Hill, 2009.
Nishioka K, Fujishima K, Kobayashi H, Mizuno Y, Okuma Y. An extremely unusual presentation of varicella zoster viral infection of cranial nerves mimicking Garcin syndrome. Clin Neurol Neurosurg 2006 Dec;108(8):772–774.
Alapatt JP, Premkumar S, Vasudevan RC. Garcin's syndrome—a case report. Surg Neurol 2007 Feb;67(2):184–185.

Gerstmann Syndrome

- Organs Involved
  - Angular gyrus, parietal lobe, dominant hemisphere of brain
- Diagnostic Characteristics
  - Finger agnosia: inability to name different fingers on the hand
  - Dysgraphia/agraphia: deficiency in ability to write
  - Dyscalculia/acalculia: difficulty in learning mathematics
  - Right-left confusion: inability to differentiate right from left
- Associated Abnormalities
  - Aphasia in adults with stroke involving the dominant parietal lobe
  - Constructional apraxia in children with developmental Gerstmann syndrome; an inability to copy simple drawings
- Treatment
  - Occupational and speech therapies
  - Calculators and word processors
- Prognosis
  - Improvement over time. Learn to adjust to deficits

References

Original:
Gerstmann J. Fingeragnosie: Eine umschriebene storung der orientierung am eigenen korper. Wiener Klinische Wochenschrift. 1924;37:1010–1012. (Translation in Archives of Neurology, Chicago. 1971;24:475–476)

Review and Case Reports:
Critchley M. The enigma of Gerstmann's syndrome. Brain 1966;89(2):183–198.
Miller CJ, Hynd GW. Whatever happened to developmental Gerstmann's syndrome? Links to other pediatric, genetic, and neurodevelopmental syndromes. J Child Neurol 2004 Apr;19(4):282–289.
Reeve R, Humberstone J. Five- to 7-year-olds' finger agnosia and calculation abilities. Front Psychol 2011;2:359.

Goldenhar Syndrome
(alt: Oculo-auriculo-vertebral (OAV) syndrome)

- Organs Involved
  - First and second branchial arches. Ears, face, eyes, mandible, skeleton, heart, renal, gastric, brain, nerve

- Diagnostic Characteristics
  - Microtia – partially formed or absent ear pinna
  - Asymmetric mouth, facial nerve paralysis
  - Absent eye or ocular dermoid
  - Vertebral scoliosis, unstable cervical spine

- Associated Abnormalities
  - Hearing and vision impairment
  - Dental and palatal anomalies
  - Congenital heart defect
  - Unilateral underdeveloped or absent intestine, kidney, lung
  - Mental retardation, microcephaly

- Differential Diagnosis
  - Hemifacial microsomia: facial asymmetry without internal organ and vertebral anomalies

- Cause
  - Unknown, multifactorial, possible genetic component, autosomal dominant or recessive, usually sporadic, male:female ratio 2:1
  - Maldevelopment in late first trimester
  - Children of Gulf war veterans susceptible, but relationship not proven

- Treatment
  - Surgical reconstruction
  - Hearing aids and glasses
  - Multidisciplinary care

References

Original:
Goldenhar M. Associations malformatives de l'oeil et de l'oreille, en particulier le syndrome dermoide epibulbaire-appendices auriculaires-fistula auris congenital et ses relations avec la dysostose mandibulo-faciale. Journal de genetique humaine., Geneve. 1952;1:243–282.

Review and Case Reports:
Touliatou V, Fryssira H, Mavrou A, Kanavakis E, Kitsiou-Tzeli S. Clinical manifestations in 17 Greek patients with Goldenhar syndrome. Genet Couns 2006;17(3):359–370.

Gorlin Syndrome
(alt: Nevoid basal cell carcinoma syndrome (NBCCS))

- Organs Involved
  - Skin, nervous system, eyes, endocrine system, bones
- Diagnostic Characteristics
  - Multiple basal cell carcinomas of skin
  - Odontogenic keratocysts in mandible
  - Rib and vertebrae anomalies
  - Intracranial calcifications, falx cerebri
  - Kyphoscoliosis, bifid ribs
  - Facies: frontal bossing, hypertelorism, prognathism, cleft lip and palate
  - First-degree relative with NBCCS
- Associated Abnormalities
  - Nervous system: blindness, deafness, mental retardation, seizures
  - Macrocephaly
  - Medulloblastoma in children usually <2 years old
  - Congenital malformations: coloboma, microphthalmia
  - Polydactyly
- Genetics
  - Autosomal dominant inheritance
  - Caused by mutations in the PTCH gene on chromosome 9q

References

Original:
Gorlin R, Goltz R. Multiple nevoid basal-cell epithelioma, jaw cysts, and bifid rib. A syndrome. N Engl J Med 1960;262(18):908–912.

Review and Case Reports:
Kimonis V, Goldstein A, Pastakia B, et al. Clinical manifestations in 105 persons with nevoid basal cell carcinoma syndrome. Am J Med Genet 1997;69(3):299–308.

Gradenigo Syndrome

- ■ Organs Involved
  - Petrous temporal bone, sixth cranial nerve
- ■ Diagnostic Characteristics
  - Otitis media and mastoiditis involving petrous apex bone
  - Cr VI nerve lateral gaze palsy
  - Retro-orbital pain (area supplied by ophthalmic branch of trigeminal Vth Cr nerve)
- ■ Associated Abnormalities
  - Bell's palsy, when VIIth nerve also involved
  - Excessive lacrimation
  - Reduced corneal sensitivity

References

Original:
Gradenigo G. Sulla leptomeningite circonscritta e sulla paralisi dell' abducenta di origine otitica. Giornale dell'Accademia di Medicina di Torino. 1904;10:59–84.

Review and Case Reports:
Sherman SC, Buchanan A. Gradenigo syndrome: a case report and review of a rare complication of otitis media. J Emerg Med 2004 Oct;27(3):253–256.
Ibrahim M, Shah G, Parmar H. Diffusion-weighted MRI identifies petrous apex abscess in Gradenigo syndrome. J Neuroophthalmol 2010 Mar;30(1):34–36.

Greig Cephalopolysyndactyly Syndrome
(alt: GCPS)

- **Organs Involved**
  - Head, eyes, hands, feet, brain
- **Diagnostic Characteristics**
  - Polydactyly
  - Syndactyly
  - Hypertelorism
  - Macrocephaly, high prominent forehead
  - Antenatal diagnosis; ultrasound for polydactyly; amniocentesis
- **Associated Abnormalities**
  - Craniosynostosis
  - Agenesis of corpus callosum
  - Developmental delay, mental retardation
  - Diaphragmatic hernia
  - Leukemia and gliomas
- **Genetics**
  - Mutations in the GLI3 gene on chromosome 7
  - Autosomal dominant inheritance
- **Differential Diagnosis**
  - Acrocallosal syndrome
  - Gorlin syndrome
  - Carpenter syndrome
  - Teebi syndrome

References

Original:
Greig DM. Oxycephaly. Edinb Med J 1926;33:189–218.

Review and Case Reports:
Gorlin RJ, Cohen MM Jr, Hennekam RCM. Greig cephalopolysyndactyly syndrome. In Syndromes of the Head and Neck, 4th edition. Eds: Gorlin RJ, Cohen MM Jr, Hennekam RCM. New York: Oxford University Press 2001:995–996.
Baraitser M, Winter RM, Brett EM. Greig cephalopolysyndactyly: report of 13 individuals in three families. Clin Genet 1983;24:257–265.
Biesecker LG. The Greig cephalopolysyndactyly syndrome. Orphanet Jr Rare Diseases 2008; 3:10–18.

Guillain-Barre Syndrome
(alt: Acute idiopathic polyradiculoneuritis)

- Organs Involved
  - Peripheral nerves, limb muscles, lower cranial nerves, face, bulbar muscles, respiratory muscles, sensory nerves, autonomic nervous system
- Diagnostic Characteristics
  - Initial symmetrical weakness of lower limbs
  - Progression of weakness upwards in hours or days. Areflexia
  - Involvement of arms, facial, and bulbar muscles
  - Dysphagia, respiratory difficulties
  - Eye muscles spared
- Additional Abnormalities
  - Sensory loss (position sense)
  - Autonomic dysfunction (orthostatic hypotension, cardiac arrhythmias)
  - Hyponatremia
  - CSF protein 100–1000 mg/dL; albuminocytologic dissociation
- Cause
  - Autoimmune disease, immune response to foreign antigens (infection): Campylobacter jejuni, cytomegalovirus, influenza virus
- Diagnostic Tests and Supportive Findings
  - CSF elevated protein level
  - EMG and NCS conduction slowing and block
- Treatment
  - Plasmapheresis or IV immunoglobulin
  - Physiotherapy rehabilitation
- Prognosis
  - Complete recovery 80 % within months to a year. Death rate at 2–3 %
  - 5–10 % relapse rate (chronic inflammatory demyelinating polyneuropathy)

References

Original:
Guillain G, Barre JA, Strohl A. Sur un syndrome de radiculonevrite avec hyperalbuminose du liquid cephalo-rachidien sans reaction cellulaire. Remarques sur les caracteres cliniques et graphiques des reflexes tendineux. Bulletins et memoires de la Societe des Medecins des Hopitaux de Paris. 1916;40:1462–1470.

Review and Case Reports:
Lin JJ, Hsia SH, Wang HS, et al. Clinical variants of Guillain-Barre syndrome in children. Pediatr Neurol 2012 Aug;47(2):91–96.
Hughes RA, Wijdicks EF, Barohn R, et al. Practice parameter: immunotherapy for Guillain-Barre syndrome: report of the Quality Standards Subcommittee of the American Academy of Neurology. Neurology 2003 Sept;61(6):736–740.

H

Hallermann-Streiff
Syndrome – HHH Syndrome

Hallermann-Streiff Syndrome
HARP Syndrome
Haw River Syndrome
Heerfordt Syndrome
Herpes Zoster Oticus Syndrome
Hopkins Syndrome
Holmes-Adie Syndrome
Horner Syndrome
HHH Syndrome

J.G. Millichap, *Neurological Syndromes: A Clinical Guide to Symptoms and Diagnosis*, DOI 10.1007/978-1-4614-7786-0_8,
© Springer Science+Business Media New York 2013

Hallermann-Streiff Syndrome
(alt: Francois dyscephalic syndrome)

- Organs Involved
  - Eyes, face, head, brain
- Diagnostic Characteristics
  - Multiple congenital abnormalities
  - Brachycephaly, frontal bossing, delayed closure of fontanelles and sutures
  - Birdlike facies with beaked nose and micrognathia, dental anomalies
  - Microphthalmia, congenital cataracts, glaucoma
  - Dwarfism, hypotrichosis
  - Mental retardation
- Genetics and Etiology
  - May be associated with GJA1 gene mutation, usually sporadic
  - Possibly autosomal recessive inheritance
  - Affects both sexes

References

Original:

Hallermann W. Vogelgesicht und cataracta congenita. Klinische Monatsblatter fur Augenheilkunde, Stuttgart. 1948;113:315–318.

Streiff EB. Dysmorphie mandibulo-faciale (tete d'oiseau) et alterations oculaires. Ophthalmologica, Basel. 1950;120:79–83.

Francois J. A new syndrome: dyscephalia with bird face and dental anomalies, nanism, hypotrichosis, cutaneous atrophy, microphthalmia and congenital cataract. Arch Ophthalmol, Chicago. 1958;60:842.

Review and Case Reports:

Hou JW. Hallermann-Streiff syndrome associated with small cerebellum, endocrinopathy and increased chromosomal breakage. Acta Paediatr 2003 Jul;92(7):869–871.

Sigirci A, Alkan A, Bicak U, Yakinci C. Hallermann-Streiff syndrome associated with complete agenesis of the corpus callosum. J Child Neurol 2005 Aug;20(8):691–693.

HARP Syndrome

- Organs Involved
  - Blood, retina, globus pallidum

- Diagnostic Characteristics
  - Hypoprebetalipoproteinemia
  - Acanthocytosis
  - Retinitis pigmentosa
  - Pallidal degeneration

- Associated Abnormalities
  - MRI "eye-of-the-tiger" sign
  - Night blindness
  - Dysarthria, dysphagia, orobuccolingual dystonia
  - Mental retardation

- Differential Diagnosis
  - Pantothenate kinase-associated neurodegeneration (PKAN, formerly Hallervorden-Spatz syndrome). HARP now considered part of the PKAN disease spectrum (Ching KH et al. 2002)
  - Bassen-Kornzweig syndrome

- Genetics
  - HARP is allelic with PKAN. PKAN is autosomal recessive.
  - Mutant PANK2 gene at chromosome locus 20p13.

- Treatment
  - Iron-chelating agents
  - Vitamins, pantothenate (PANK2 enzyme substrate), coenzyme Q

- Prognosis
  - Progressive neurodegeneration. Survival rate 11 years

References

Original:
Hallervorden J, Spatz H. 1922

Review and Case Reports:
Orrell RW, Amrolia PJ, Heald A, et al. Acanthocytosis, retinitis pigmentosa, and pallidal degeneration: a report of three patients, including the second reported case with hypoprebetalipoproteinemia (HARP syndrome). Neurology 1995 Mar;45(3 Pt 1):487–492
Ching KH, Westaway SK, Gitschier J, Higgins JJ, Hayflick SJ. HARP syndrome is allelic with pantothenate kinase-associated neurodegeneration. Neurology 2002 Jun 11;58(11):1673–1674.

Haw River Syndrome
(alt: Dentatorubral-pallidoluysian atrophy (DRPLA), Naito-Oyanagi disease)

- Organs Involved
  - Dentate nucleus, globus pallidus, centrum semiovale, posterior spinal columns

- Diagnostic Characteristics
  - Ataxia
  - Seizures, myoclonus epilepsy
  - Choreiform movements, cervical dystonia
  - Loss of vibration and position sense
  - Progressive dementia
  - Juvenile, early adult and late adult onset

- Associated Abnormalities
  - Neuronal loss of dentate nucleus
  - Calcification of globus pallidus
  - Neuroaxonal dystrophy of nuclei gracilis and cuneatus
  - Demyelination of centrum semiovale
  - Marked brain atrophy, neuronal intranuclear inclusions

- Differential Diagnosis
  - Huntington's disease
  - Spinocerebellar ataxias
  - Progressive myoclonus epilepsy, Unverricht-Lundborg disease
  - Neuroaxonal dystrophy

- Genetics
  - Autosomal dominant. More frequent in Japanese population
  - Expansion of a CAG repeat encoding a polyglutamine region of the atrophin 1 gene on chromosome 12p13.3. Displays anticipation
  - Named after the hometown (Haw River, North Carolina) of the first recorded member of the affected family reported (Farmer et al. 1989)

- Prognosis
  - Death at 15–25 years after onset

References

Original:
Farmer TW, Wingfield MS, Lynch SA, et al. Ataxia, chorea, seizures, and dementia. Pathologic features of a newly defined familial disorder. Arch Neurol 1989 Jul;46(7):774–779.

Review and Case Reports:
Burke JR, Wingfield MS, Lewis KE, et al. The Haw River syndrome: dentatorubro-pallidoluysian atrophy (DRPLA) in an African-American family. Nat Genet 1994 Aug;7(4):521–524.

Heerfordt Syndrome
(alt: Waldenstrom's uveoparotitis)

- Organs Involved
  - Parotid glands, eyes, facial nerve, and muscle
- Diagnostic Characteristics
  - Parotid gland enlargement, fever, uveitis, and facial nerve palsy
  - Sarcoidosis with meningism, CSF pleocytosis, generalized lymphade-nopathy, skin rash

References

Original:

Heerfordt CF. Uber eine "Febris uveo-parotidea subchronica" an der glandula parotis und der uvea des auges lokalisiert und haufig mit paresen cerebrospinaler nerven kompliziert. Albrecht von Grafes Arch fur Ophthalmologie. 1909;70:254–273.

Waldenstrom JG. Some observations on uveoparotitis and allied conditions with special reference to the symptoms from the nervous system. Acta Medica Scandinavica, Stockholm. 1937;91:53–68.

Review and Case Reports:

Glocker FX, Seifert C, Lucking CH. Facial palsy in Heerfordt's syndrome: electrophysiological localization of the lesion. Muscle Nerve 1999 Sep;22(9):1279–1282.

Herpes Zoster Oticus Syndrome
(alt: Ramsay Hunt syndrome type II)

- Organs Involved
  - Geniculate ganglion, face, ear, tongue, vestibulocochlear nerve
- Diagnostic Characteristics
  - Acute facial nerve paralysis
  - Pain in the ear
  - Loss of taste, anterior 2/3rds tongue
  - Dry mouth and eyes
  - Erythematous vesicular rash in the ear canal, tongue, and hard palate
- Associated Abnormalities
  - Tinnitus, hearing loss, vertigo
- Pathophysiology
  - Shingles of the geniculate ganglion
  - Illness that suppresses the immune system
- Prevention
  - Vaccination with Zostavax chickenpox vaccine
- Prognosis
  - Complete facial recovery in 75 % if treatment with prednisone and acyclovir started within first 3 days of onset. No recovery of hearing
  - Persistent facial paralysis in 50 % when treatment delayed

References

Original:
Hunt JR. On herpetic inflammations of the geniculate ganglion: a new syndrome and its complications. J Nerv Ment Dis 1907;34(2):73–96.

Review and Case Reports:
Murakami S, Hato N, Horiuchi J, Honda N, Gyo K, Yanagihara N. Treatment of Ramsay Hunt syndrome with acyclovir-prednisone: significance of early diagnosis and treatment. Ann Neurol 1997;41(3):353–357.

Hopkins Syndrome
(alt: Poliomyelitis-like asthmatic amyotrophy)

- Organs Involved
  - Spinal cord anterior horn cells, muscles, lungs

- Diagnostic Characteristics
  - Asthma exacerbation with viral infection (HSV type I, *Mycoplasma pneumoniae*)
  - Poliomyelitis-like, lower motor neuron paralysis (asthmatic asymmetrical amyotrophy)

- Prognosis
  - Poor, persistent weakness

References

Original:
Hopkins IJ, Shield LK. Poliomyelitis-like illness associated with asthma in childhood. Lancet 1974;1:76.
Hopkins IJ. A new syndrome: Poliomyelitis-like illness associated with acute asthma in childhood. Aust Paediatr J 1974;10:273–276.

Review and Case Reports:
Nihei K, Naitoh H, Ikeda K. Poliomyelitis-like syndrome following asthmatic attack (Hopkins syndrome). Pediatr Neurol 1987 May-Jun;3(3):166–168.
Bailey R, Johnson EW. Asthmatic amyotrophy. Three cases. Am J Phys Med Rehabil 1991 Dec;70(6):332–334.
Arita J, Nakae Y, Matsushima H, Maekawa K. Hopkins syndrome: T2-weighted high intensity of anterior horn on spinal MR imaging. Pediatr Neurol 1995 Oct;13(3):263–265.
Acharya AB, Lakhani PK. Hopkins syndrome associated with Mycoplasma infection. Pediatr Neurol 1997 Jan;16(1):54–55.

Holmes-Adie Syndrome
(alt: Adie syndrome; Ross syndrome)

■ Organs Involved
  • Eye, pupillary parasympathetic innervation, muscle reflex

■ Diagnostic Characteristics
  • Anisocoria. Dilated pupil that does not constrict quickly in response to light (Adie pupil) and impaired accommodation
  • Loss of deep tendon reflexes
  • Excessive sweating, autonomic neuropathy, orthostatic hypotension
  • Affects younger women (3:1 female preponderance), average age 30–40 years, unilateral in 80 % cases

■ Causes
  • Damage to the ciliary ganglion that normally controls pupil constriction
  • Peripheral neuropathy that causes areflexia
  • Viral or bacterial infection suspected

References

Original:
Adie WJ. Tonic pupils and absent tendon reflexes. A benign disorder *sui generis*; its complete and incomplete forms. Brain 1932;55:98.

Review and Case Reports:
Ropper AH. Samuels MA. Eds Adams and Victor's Principles of Neurology, ninth edition; New York, McGraw Hill, 2009.
Nolano M, Provitera V, Donadio V, et al. Ross syndrome: a lesson from a monozygotic twin pair. Neurology 2013;80:417–418.

Horner Syndrome
(alt: Oculosympathetic palsy)

- Organs Involved
  - Oculosympathetic nervous system: (1) central involving hypothalamospinal tract and cord, (2) preganglionic with compression of sympathetic chain, and (3) postganglionic at level of internal carotid and cavernous sinus

- Diagnostic Characteristics
  - Ptosis
  - Miosis
  - Enophthalmos
  - Anhidrosis of affected side of face

- Associated Abnormalities
  - Heterochromia in congenital Horner syndrome

- Acquired Causes
  - Lateral medullary syndrome, vertebral artery, or PICA stroke
  - Trauma at base of neck
  - Middle ear infection
  - Pancoast tumor, bronchogenic carcinoma at apex of lung
  - Aortic aneurysm
  - Neurofibromatosis type 1
  - Thyroid carcinoma
  - Multiple sclerosis
  - Klumpke paralysis
  - Cavernous sinus thrombosis
  - Syringomyelia
  - During migraine attack

- Differential Diagnosis
  - Oculomotor third nerve palsy has a dilated pupil, and ptosis is severe.
  - Horner syndrome has constricted pupil, and ptosis is mild and partial.

- Test for Horner Syndrome
  - Cocaine eye drops fail to dilate the Horner pupil lacking norepinephrine.
  - A-agonist apraclonidine has increased mydriatic effect on Horner pupil.

References

Original:
Horner JF. Uber eine Form von Ptosis. Klin Monatsbl Augenheilk 1869;7:193–198.

Review and Case Reports:
Lee JH, Lee HK, Lee DH, Choi CG, Kim SJ, Suh DC. Neuroimaging strategies for three types of Horner syndrome with emphasis on anatomic location. AJR Am J Roentgenol 2007;188(1): W74-81.

HHH Syndrome
(alt: Hyperornithinemia-hyperammonemia-homocitrullinuria syndrome; ornithine translocase deficiency syndrome)

- Organs Involved
  - Liver, urea cycle disorder, central nervous system
- Diagnostic Characteristics
  - Neonatal onset (~12 % cases) at 24–48 h, with poor feeding, vomiting, hypothermia, hyperpnea
  - Infancy, childhood, and adult presentation (~88 %), with chronic neuro-cognitive deficits, developmental delay, ataxia, spastic paraparesis, learning disabilities, seizures
  - Acute encephalopathy secondary to hyperammonemic crisis
  - Chronic liver dysfunction, elevated liver transaminases, hyperammonemia, and protein intolerance
- Genetics
  - Mutations in SLC25A15 gene that encodes ORNT1 (mitochondrial ornithine transporter 1) involved in the urea cycle and the ornithine degradation pathway
  - Metabolic diagnostic triad: hyperornithinemia, hyperammonemia, homocitrullinuria
  - Autosomal recessive inheritance
- Treatment
  - Control hyperammonemic episodes by reducing protein intake.
  - Protein-restricted diet.
  - Avoid protein supplements, prolonged fasting, IV steroids, valproic acid.

References

Early:
Hommes FA, Roesel RA, Metoki K, Hartlage PL, Dyken PR. Studies on a case of HHH-syndrome. Neuropediatrics 1986 Feb;17(1):48–52.

Review and Case Reports:
Scriver C, Beaudet al, Valle D, et al. The Online Metabolic and Molecular Bases of Inherited Disease. New York; McGraw-Hill, 2007; chap 83.
Camacho J, Rioseco-Camacho N. Hyperornithinemia-Hyperammonemia-Homocitrullinuria syndrome. In GeneReviews edited by Pagon RA, Bird TD, Dolan CR, et al. Seattle (WA): University of Washington. Seattle, 1993-
Salvi S, Santorelli FM, Bertini E, et al. Clinical and molecular findings in hyperornithinemia-hyperammonemia-homocitrullinuria syndrome. Neurology 2001 Sep 11;57(5):911–914.

I

Isaacs Syndrome

Isaacs Syndrome

J.G. Millichap, *Neurological Syndromes: A Clinical Guide to Symptoms and Diagnosis*, DOI 10.1007/978-1-4614-7786-0_9,
© Springer Science+Business Media New York 2013

Isaacs Syndrome
(alt: Immune-mediated neuromyotonia; acquired neuromyotonia)

- Organs Involved
  - Muscles, nerves
- Diagnostic Characteristics
  - Muscle cramps, stiffness, especially in calves, trunk, and sometimes neck and face, due to hyperexcitability of peripheral nerve, including autonomic nerve
  - Myotonia-like symptoms (slow relaxation)
  - Hyperidrosis
  - Myokymia, fasciculations
  - Exercise intolerance
  - Onset between 15 and 60 years old
- Associated Abnormalities
  - Spontaneous, rapid discharges of single motor-unit potentials and myokymic and neuromyotonic discharges on EMG
  - An antibody-mediated potassium channel disorder (channelopathy), relieved by Na channel blocker and immunotherapy
  - Sometimes associated with neoplasm, especially thymoma
- Differential Diagnosis
  - Types of neuromyotonia: acquired (chronic, monophasic – postinfection, and relapsing remitting), paraneoplastic, hereditary
  - Morvan syndrome
  - Amyotrophic lateral sclerosis

References

Original:
Isaacs H. A syndrome of continuous muscle-fibre activity. J Neurol Neurosurg Psychiatry 1961 Nov;24(4):319–325.

Review and Case Reports:
Gonzales G, Barros G, Russi ME, Nunez A, Scavone C. Acquired neuromyotonia in childhood: case report and review. Pediatr Neurol 2008 Jan;38(1):61–63.
Arimura K, Watanabe O. Immune-mediated neuromyotonia (Isaacs' syndrome)—clinical aspects and pathomechanism. Brain Nerve 2010 Apr;62(4):401–410.

J

Jackson Syndrome – Juberg-Marsidi Syndrome

Jackson Syndrome
Jackson-Weiss Syndrome
Jacobsen Syndrome
Janz Syndrome
Jervell and Lange-Nielsen Syndrome
Joubert Syndrome
Juberg-Marsidi Syndrome

J.G. Millichap, *Neurological Syndromes: A Clinical Guide to Symptoms and Diagnosis*, DOI 10.1007/978-1-4614-7786-0_10,
© Springer Science+Business Media New York 2013

Jackson Syndrome
(alt: Hughlings Jackson syndrome)

- Organs Involved
  - Tegmentum of medulla oblongata, cranial nerves X and XII
- Diagnostic Characteristics
  - Ipsilateral paralysis of soft palate, pharynx, larynx, and ipsilateral paralysis and hemiatrophy of the tongue
  - Contralateral hemianesthesia (same as Avellis syndrome)
- Causes
  - Infarct or tumor

References

Original:
Jackson JH. In: Clinical Lectures and Reports by the Medical and Surgical Staff of the London Hospital, London 1864;1:368. On a case of paralysis of the tongue from haemorrhage in the medulla oblongata.
Idem. The Lancet, London, 1872;2:770–773.
Idem. Paralysis of tongue, palate, and vocal cord. The Lancet, 1886;1:689–690.
MacKenzie S. Two cases of associated paralysis of the tongue, soft palate, and vocal cord on the same side. Transactions of the Clinical Society of London, 1886;19:317–319.

Case Report:
Chang D, Cho SH. Medial medullary infarction with contralateral glossoplegia. J Neurol Neurosurg Psychiatry 2005 Jun;76(6):888.
See Brainstem syndromes. Table and individual syndromes

Jackson-Weiss Syndrome

■ Organs Involved
  • Skull, feet

■ Diagnostic Characteristics
  • Craniosynostosis, bulging forehead
  • Hypertelorism, midface hypoplasia
  • Premature fusion of foot bones, enlarged big toes

■ Genetics and Etiology
  • Mutations in the FGFR2 gene on chromosome 10
  • Autosomal dominant inheritance

■ Differential Diagnosis of FGFR-Craniosynostosis Syndromes
  • Pfeiffer, Apert, Crouzon, Beare-Stevenson, and Muenke syndromes

References

Original:
Jackson CE, Weiss L, Reynolds WA, Forman TF, Peterson JA. Craniosynostosis, midfacial hypo-plasia and foot abnormalities: an autosomal dominant phenotype in a large Amish kindred. J Pedaitr 1976 Jun;88(6):963–968.

Review and Case Reports:
Robin NH, Falk MJ, Haldeman-Englert CR. FGFR-related craniosynostosis syndromes. In: Pagon RA, Bird TD, Dolan CR, Stephens K, Adam MP. Editors. GeneReviews [Internet]. Seattle (WA): University of Washington, Seattle; 1993–1998 Oct 20 [updated 2011 Jun 07].
Heike C, Seto M, Hing A, et al. Century of Jackson-Weiss syndrome: further definition of clinical and radiographic findings in "lost" descendants of the original kindred. Am J Med Genet 2001;100(4):315–324.

Jacobsen Syndrome
(alt: 11q deletion disorder)

- **Organs Involved**
  - Brain, face, heart, blood, extremities

- **Diagnostic Characteristics**
  - Intellectual disabilities
  - Facial/skeletal dysplasia, short stature
  - Trigonocephaly, wide-set eyes
  - Retrognathia
  - Low-set, misshapen ears; short upturned nose; anteverted nostrils
  - Camptodactyly (upward curvature of pinkie and ring fingers)
  - Large great toes/hammertoes
  - Heart defects, renal defects, cryptorchidism
  - Thrombocytopenia

- **Differential Diagnosis**
  - Turner syndrome
  - Noonan syndrome
  - Acquired thrombocytopenia

- **Genetics**
  - Partial deletion of long arm of chromosome 11, including band 11q24.1
  - Female/male ratio 2:1
  - Mainly sporadic, occasionally familial

References

Original:
Jacobsen P, Hauge M, Henningsen K, Hobolth N, Mikkelsen M, Philip JK. An (11.21) translocation in four generations with chromosome 11 abnormalities in the offspring. A clinical, cytoge-
netical, and gene marker study. Hum Hered 1973;23(6):568–585.

Review Article:
Mattina T, Perrotta CS, Grossfeld P. Jacobsen syndrome. Orphanet Jrnl Rare Dis 2009;4:9–23.

Janz Syndrome
(alt: Juvenile myoclonic epilepsy (JME))

- Organs Involved
  - Shoulders, arms, brain

- Diagnostic Characteristics
  - Onset at 12–18 years old
  - Sudden jerks of shoulders and arms, on awakening or while falling asleep
  - Generalized tonic-clonic seizures, triggered by sleep deprivation
  - Absence seizures

- Associated Abnormalities
  - Interictal EEG shows bilateral, symmetrical, synchronous, and diffuse polyspike and slow wave complexes at 4–6 Hz/s.
  - Positive family history for epilepsy in 50 % cases.
  - Neurologic exam and imaging studies are normal.

- Genetics
  - Mutations of several genes (CACNB4, GABRA1, etc.) located on the short arm of chromosome 6

- Treatment
  - Avoid sleep deprivation, early awakening, alcohol, and flickering lights.
  - Medication must be continued without interruption for a lifetime.

References

Original:
Janz D, Christian W. Impulsiv-petit mal. Deutsche Zeitschrift fur Nervenheilkunde 1957;176: 346–386.

Review and Case Reports:
Janz D. The idiopathic generalized epilepsies of adolescence with childhood and juvenile age of onset. Epilepsia 1997;39:4–11.
Wandschneider B, Thompson PJ, Vollmar C, Koepp MJ. Frontal lobe function and structure in juvenile myoclonic epilepsy: a comprehensive review of neuropsychological and imaging data. Epilepsia 2012 Dec;53(12):2091–2098.

Jervell and Lange-Nielsen Syndrome
(alt: Cardioauditory syndrome of Jervell and Lange-Nielsen; Surdo Cardiac syndrome; long QT syndrome 1)

- Organs Involved
  - Auditory nerve, inner ear, heart
- Diagnostic Characteristics
  - Congenital profound sensorineural hearing loss
  - Long QT interval, usually >500 ms, associated with ventricular tachycardia and fibrillation which may result in syncope or sudden death
- Associated Abnormalities
  - Syncopal episodes during periods of stress, exercise, or fright.
  - Iron-deficient anemia and elevated levels of gastrin.
  - Cardiac events in 50 % cases before 3 years of age.
  - Mortality rate: if untreated, >50 % die before age 15 years.
- Genetics
  - Mutations in either KCNQ1 or KCNE1 gene
  - Autosomal recessive inheritance
- Management
  - Cochlear implantation to treat hearing loss
  - Beta-adrenergic blockers for long QT interval
  - Treatment of iron-deficiency anemia
  - Special precautions during anesthesia
  - Avoid drugs that prolong the QT interval

References

Original:
Jervell A, Lange-Nielsen F. Congenital deaf-mutism, functional heart disease with prolongation of the Q-T interval and sudden death. Am Heart J 1957;54:59–68.

Review and Case Reports:
Schwartz PJ, Spazzolini C, Crotti L, et al. The Jervell and Lange-Nielsen syndrome: natural history, molecular basis, and clinical outcome. Circulation 2006;1132:783–790.
Tranebjaerg L, Samson RA, Green GE. Jervell and Lange-Nielsen syndrome. In: Pagon RA, Bird TD, Dolan GR, et al. editors. GeneReviews [Internet], Seattle (WA): University of Washington, Seattle; 1993–2002; Last update Oct 4, 2012.

Joubert Syndrome

- Organs Involved
  - Cerebellar vermis, brainstem
- Diagnostic Characteristics
  - Ataxia, agenesis of cerebellar vermis
  - Episodic hyperpnea, sleep apnea
  - Irregular jerky eye movements
  - Mental retardation
- Associated Abnormalities
  - MRI "molar tooth sign"
  - Retinal coloboma, retinitis pigmentosa
  - Polydactyly
  - Cleft lip or palate, tongue abnormalities
  - Seizures
- Genetics
  - Multiple mutated genes
  - A ciliopathy

References

Original:
Joubert M, Eisenring JJ, Robb JP, Anderman F. Familial agenesis of the cerebellar vermis. A syndrome of episodic hyperpnea, abnormal eye movements, ataxia, and retardation. Neurology 1969;19(9):813–825.

Reviews:
Saraiva JM, Baraitser M. Joubert syndrome: a review. Am J Med Genet 1992;43(4):726–731.
Badano JL, Norimasa Mitsuma PL, Beales NK. The ciliopathies: An emerging class of human genetic disorders. Annual Review of Genomics and Human Genetics 2006 Sep;7:125–148.

Juberg-Marsidi Syndrome

- Organs Involved
  - Brain, muscle, skeleton, genitalia

- Diagnostic Characteristics
  - Microcephaly
  - Sensorineural deafness
  - Short stature, growth retardation
  - Ocular anomalies, flat nasal bridge
  - Severe mental retardation
  - Hypogonadism, hypogenitalia
  - Delayed milestones
  - Hypotonia, muscle weakness

- Genetics
  - X-linked recessive inheritance
  - Mutations of the ATRX gene on the long arm of the X-chromosome (Xq12-q21)

- Differential Diagnosis
  - Carpenter syndrome
  - Smith-Fineman-Myers syndrome

References

Original:
Juberg RC, Marsidi I. A new form of X-linked mental retardation with growth retardation, deafness, and microgenitalism. Am J Hum Genet 1980 Sep;32(5):714–722.

Review and Case Reports:
Saugier-Veber P, Abadie V, Moncla A, et al. The Juberg-Marsidi syndrome maps to the proximal long arm of the X chromosome (Xq12-q21). Am J Hum Genet 1993 Jun;52(6):1040–1045.

K

Kabuki Syndrome – Kocher-Debre-Semelaigne Syndrome

Kabuki Syndrome
Kallmann Syndrome
Kearns-Sayre Syndrome (KSS)
Kinsbourne Syndrome
Kjellin Syndrome
Kleefstra Syndrome
Klein-Levin Syndrome
Klinefelter Syndrome
Klippel-Feil Syndrome
Klippel-Trenaunay-Weber Syndrome
Kluver-Bucy Syndrome
Kocher-Debre-Semelaigne Syndrome

J.G. Millichap, *Neurological Syndromes: A Clinical Guide to Symptoms and Diagnosis*, DOI 10.1007/978-1-4614-7786-0_11,
© Springer Science+Business Media New York 2013

Kabuki Syndrome
(alt: Niikawa-Kuroki syndrome)

- Organs Involved
  - Face, skeleton, joints, ears, heart, urinary tract
- Diagnostic Characteristics
  - Long eyelids
  - Broad, depressed nasal tip
  - Prominent earlobes
  - Cleft or high arched palate
  - Scoliosis, short fifth finger
  - Heart defects
- Associated Abnormalities
  - Mild to moderate intellectual disability
  - Unusually sociable, happy disposition
  - Focal seizures, fronto-central localization
  - Characteristic EEG pattern, fronto-central biphasic spikes and slow wave
  - MRI T2 hyperintensities in deep brain nuclei with tremor in one report and dilated vein of Galen in another
- Genetics
  - Autosomal dominant or X-linked recessive inheritance
  - Two-thirds of cases have mutation in the MLL2 gene

References

Original:
Kuroki Y, Suzuki Y, Chyo H, Hata A, Matsui I. A new malformation syndrome of long palpebral fissures, large ears, depressed nasal tip, and skeletal anomalies associated with postnatal dwarfism and mental retardation. J Pediatr 1981 Oct;99(4):570–573.

Review and Case Reports:
Lodi M, Chifari R, Parazzini C, et al. Seizures and EEG pattern in Kabuki syndrome. Brain Dev 2010 Nov;32(10):829–834.
Grunseich C, Fishbein TM, Berkowitz F, Shamim EA. Tremor and deep brain nuclei hyperintensities in Kabuki syndrome. Pediatr Neurol 2010 Aug;43(2):148–150.
Sannchez-Carpintero R, Herranz A, Reynoso C, Zubieta JL. Dilated vein of Galen in Kabuki syndrome. Brain Dev 2012 Jan;34(1):76–79.

Kallmann Syndrome
(alt: Hypogonadotropic hypogonadism (HH) with anosmia syndrome)

- Organs Involved
  - Hypothalamus, pituitary, olfactory bulbs, eyes, skull

- Diagnostic Characteristics
  - Idiopathic hypogonadotropic hypogonadism
  - Congenital hypothalamic dysfunction
  - Pituitary hypogonadism, eunuchoidism
  - Small genitalia, absent pubic hair
  - Anosmia/hyposmia
  - Degeneration of olfactory bulbs

- Associated Abnormalities
  - Retinitis pigmentosa, color blindness
  - Midline cranial defects, synkinesis
  - Renal agenesis
  - Hypertension, obesity
  - Diabetes mellitus
  - Mental retardation

- Genetics
  - Autosomal dominant, some cases recessive or X-linked
  - Males affected more often than females
  - Mutations in several genes, including CHD7 and WDR11

References

Original:
Maestre de San Juan A. Teratolagia: falta total de los nervios olfactorios con anosmia en un individuo en quien existia una atrofia congenital de los testiculos y miembro viril. El siglo medico, Madrid 1856;211.
Kallmann FJ, Schonfeld WA, Barrera SE. The genetic aspects of primary eunuchoidism. Am J Mental Deficiency 1943–1944;48:203–236.
De Morsier G. Median cranioencephalic dysraphias and olfactogenital dysplasia. World Neurology, Minneapolis 1962;3:485–506.

Review and Case Reports:
Kaplan JD, Berstein JA, Kwan A, Hudgins L. Clues to an early diagnosis of Kallmann syndrome. Am J Med Genet A 2010 Nov;152A(11):2796–2801.
Kim HG, Layman LC. The role of CHD7 and the newly identified WDR11 gene in patients with idiopathic hypogonadotropic hypogonadism and Kallmann syndrome. Mol Cell Endocrinol 2011 Oct 22;346(1–2):74–83.
Gutierrez-Amavizca BE, Figuera LE, Orozco-Castellanos R. Current genetic issues and phenotypic variants in Kallmann syndrome. Rev Med Inst Mex Seguro Soc 2012 Mar-Apr;50(2): 157–161.

Kearns-Sayre Syndrome (KSS)
(alt: Oculocraniosomatic neuromuscular disease with ragged red fibers)

- Organs Involved
  - Eye muscles, cerebellum, CSF, mitochondria, heart

- Diagnostic Characteristics
  - Chronic progressive external ophthalmoplegia (CPEO)
  - Ptosis, unilateral, later bilateral
  - Pigmentary retinopathy (salt and pepper appearance), at macula
  - Cardiac conduction abnormalities, AV block

- Associated Abnormalities
  - Cerebellar ataxia
  - Proximal muscle weakness, first unilateral, later bilateral
  - Deafness
  - Diabetes mellitus, growth hormone deficiency, hypoparathyroidism
  - Elevated CSF protein (>100 mg/dl), elevated blood lactate

- Genetics
  - Deletions in mitochondrial DNA, maternal transmission
  - Ragged red fibers in orbicularis oculi muscle biopsy

- Treatment
  - Coenzyme Q10 supplements
  - Pacemaker implant
  - Endocrine screening

References

Original:
Kearns TP, Sayre GP. Retinitis pigmentosa, external ophthalmoplegia, and complete heart block: unusual syndrome with histologic study in one of two cases. AMA Arch Ophthalmol 1956 Aug;60(2):280–289.
Kearns TP. External ophthalmoplegia, pigmentary degeneration of the retina, and cardiomyopathy: A newly recognized syndrome. Trans Am Ophthalmol Soc 1965;63:559–625.

Review and Case Reports:
Lestienne P, Ponsot G. Kearns-Sayre syndrome with muscle mitochondrial DNA deletion. Lancet 1988 April;1(8590):885.
Lax NZ, Campbell GR, Reeve AK, et al. Loss of myelin-associated glycoprotein in kearns-sayre syndrome. Arch Neurol 2012 Apr;69(4):490–499.

Kinsbourne Syndrome
(alt: Opsoclonus myoclonus; dancing eyes syndrome)

- Organs Involved
  - Eyes, trunk, limbs, diaphragm, larynx, pharynx

- Diagnostic Characteristics
  - Random, high-amplitude, arrhythmic, multidirectional, involuntary conjugate eye movements
  - Focal or diffuse myoclonus, involving trunk, limbs, diaphragm, larynx, pharynx
  - Aphasia, mutism
  - Lethargy, sleep disorder
  - Maybe self-limiting when associated with viral encephalitis
  - When occurring with neuroblastoma in children, associated with anti-Hu (ANNA-!) antibodies
  - In adults, occurs with small cell lung carcinoma or breast carcinoma and associated with anti-Hu (ANNA-1) or anti-Ri (ANNA-2) antibodies

- Treatment and Prognosis
  - In children, surgery for removal of neuroblastoma and ACTH or corticosteroids. Good response usual, but may have long-term developmental and cognitive problems
  - In adults, worse prognosis for paraneoplastic syndrome cases

References

Original:
Kinsbourne M. Myoclonic encephalopathy of infants. J Neurol Neurosurg Psychiatr 1962 Aug;25(3):271–276.

Review and Case Reports:
Koh PS, Raffernsperger JG, Berry S, Larsen MB, et al. Long-term outcome in children with opsoclonus-myoclonus and ataxia and coincident neuroblastoma. J Pediatr 1994 Nov;125(5Pt 1): 712–716.

Kjellin Syndrome

- Organs Involved
  - Corpus callosum, cerebrum, retina
- Diagnostic Characteristics
  - Corpus callosum thinning
  - Hereditary progressive spastic paraplegia, onset early adulthood
  - Fundus autofluorescence and multiple retinal flecks
  - Central retina degeneration
  - Dementia
  - Peripheral neuropathy and amyotrophy
- Genetics
  - Autosomal recessive
  - Mutations in SPG11 or SPG15 genes

References

Original:
Kjellin K. Family spastic paraplegia with amyotrophy, oligophrenia, and central retinal degeneration. Arch Neurol 1959;1:133.

Review and Case Reports:
Frisch IB, Haag P, Steffen H, Weber BH, Holz FG. Kjellin's syndrome: fundus autofluorescence, angiographic, and electrophysiologic findings. Ophthalmology 2002 Aug;109(8):1484–1491.
Orien H, Melberg A, Raininko R, et al. SPG11 mutations cause Kjellin syndrome, a hereditary spastic paraplegia with thin corpus callosum and central retinal degeneration. Am J Med Genet B Neuropsychiatr Genet 2009 Oct 5;150B(7):984–992.

Kleefstra Syndrome
(alt: 9q34 deletion syndrome)

- ■ Organs Involved
  - • Face, head, eyebrows, eyes, tongue, brain

- ■ Diagnostic Characteristics
  - • Distinctive facial features: arched eyebrows joined together (synophrys), hypertelorism, midface hypoplasia, anteverted nares
  - • Prognathism
  - • Macroglossia
  - • Microcephaly, brachycephaly
  - • Hypotonia
  - • Developmental delay, learning disability, aphasia

- ■ Associated Abnormalities
  - • Structural brain abnormalities
  - • Congenital heart defects
  - • Genitourinary abnormalities
  - • Seizures
  - • Regressive behavioral phenotype: autism in childhood, apathy and catatonia in adolescence

- ■ Genetics
  - • Loss or mutations in the EHMT1 gene or deletions of chromosome 9q34.3
  - • Autosomal dominant random inheritance

References

Original:
Kleefstra T, Smidt M, Banning MJ, et al. Disruption of the gene euchromatin histone methyl transferase1 (EuHMTase1) is associated with the 9q34 subtelomeric deletion syndrome. J Med Genet 2005 Apr;42(4):299–306.

Review and Case Reports:
Willemsen MH, Vulto-van Silfhout AT, et al. Update on Kleefstra syndrome. Mol Syndromol 2012 Apr;2(3–5):202–212.

Klein-Levin Syndrome
(alt: Sleeping beauty syndrome)

- Organs Involved
  - Hypothalamus
- Diagnostic Characteristics
  - Episodic hypersomnia (~16 h a day) associated with:
  - Altered mental state
  - Cognitive impairment, confusion, hallucinations, delusions
  - Hyperphagia
  - Hypersexual behavior during episodes
- Suspected Causes
  - Malfunction of hypothalamus
  - Autoimmune disorder
  - Precipitated by infection, stress, alcohol, marijuana, or head trauma
- Differential Diagnosis
  - Diagnosis of exclusion
  - Narcolepsy
  - Metabolic problem (diabetes, hypothyroidism)
  - Multiple sclerosis
  - Cerebral tumor
  - Bipolar disorder
  - Cyclic premenstrual sleepiness in teenage girls
- Genetics
  - No known genetic markers, some familial cases
  - Adolescent males predominantly, sex ratio 3:1, Jewish males especially
  - Average age at onset 15.7 years; age range 6–59 years
- Treatment
  - Stimulants. Carbamazepine
- Prognosis
  - Median duration 8 years; 6 months between episodes (range 0.5–72 months)

References

Original:
Critchley, M, Hoffman H. The syndrome of periodic somnolence and morbid hunger (Kleine-Levin syndrome). Brit Med Jrnl, London 1942;1:137–139.
Levin M. Periodic somnolence and morbid hunger: A new syndrome. Brain, Oxford 1936;59:494–504.

Review and Case Reports:
Arnulf I, Lin L, Gadoth N, et al. Kleine-Levin syndrome: a systematic study of 108 patients. Ann Neurol 2008 Apr;63(4):482–493.

K Kabuki Syndrome – Kocher-Debre-Semelaigne Syndrome

Klinefelter Syndrome
(alt: 47,XXY or XXY syndrome)

- Organs Involved
  - Muscles, body hair, breasts, testes

- Diagnostic Characteristics
  - As children, muscle weakness and incoordination
  - At puberty, less muscular, less facial and body hair, broad hips, lack of secondary sexual characters
  - As teens, larger breasts, reduced energy level, tall stature
  - As adults, lanky build, gynecomastia, reduced fertility, microorchidism

- Associated Abnormalities
  - Increased susceptibility to autoimmune disorders, cancer, and osteoporosis
  - Learning disorders, ADHD, autism, seizures
  - Delayed motor development through infancy and childhood
  - Psychosocial morbidity – depressive anxiety

- Genetics
  - Males with Klinefelter syndrome may have a mosaic 47,XXY/46,XY karyotype.
  - The extra X chromosome is retained because of a nondisjunction event during meiosis I or II.

- Treatment
  - Testosterone to begin at puberty may normalize body shape and secondary sex characteristics but not the infertility, gynecomastia, and small testes.

References

Original:
Klinefelter HF Jr, Reifenstein EC Jr, Albright F. Syndrome characterized by gynecomastia, aspermatogenesis without a-Leydigism and increased excretion of follicle-stimulating hormone. J Clin Endocrinol Metab 1942;2(11):615–624.

Review and Case Reports:
Grosso S, Farnetani MA, Di Bartolo RM, et al. Electroencephalographic and epileptic patterns in X chromosome anomalies. J Clin Neurophysiol 2004 Jul-Aug;21(4):249–253.
Savic I. Advances in research on the neurological and neuropsychiatric phenotype of Klinefelter syndrome. Curr Opin Neurol 2012 Apr;25(2):138–143.

Klippel-Feil Syndrome

- Organs Involved
  - Cervical vertebrae

- Diagnostic Characteristics
  - Short, webbed neck
  - Decreased range of motion of cervical spine
  - Low hairline

- Types
  - I. Fusion of C2 and C3 and occipitalization of atlas
  - II. Long fusion below C2 and abnormal occipital-cervical junction
  - III. Single open interspace between two fused segments

- Associated Abnormalities
  - Scoliosis
  - Spina bifida
  - Anomalies of kidneys and ribs
  - Cleft palate
  - Short stature
  - Duane syndrome
  - Heart and other defects

- Notable Reported Cases
  - Egyptian pharaoh Tutankhamun
  - English cricketer Gladstone Small

- Genetics
  - Autosomal dominant (C2–C3 fusion) or autosomal recessive inheritance (C5–C6 fusion). Mutations in the GDF6 and GDF3 genes.
  - KFS with laryngeal malformation (Segmentation syndrome) is mapped on locus 8q22.2

- Treatment
  - Surgery to relieve cervical instability and spinal cord compression

References

Original:
Klippel M, Feil A. Un cas d'absence des vertebres cervicales. Avec cage thoracique remontant jusqu'a la base du crane (cage thoracique cervicale). Nouv Iconog Salpetriere. 1912;25: 223–250.

Review and Case Reports:
Tracy MR, Dormans JP, Kusumi K. Klippel-Feil syndrome: clinical features and current understanding of etiology. Clin Orthop Relat Res 2004 Jul;424:183–190.
McGaughran JM. Audiology abnormalities in the Klippel-Feil syndrome. Arch Dis Child 1998 Feb;79.4:352–355.

Klippel-Trenaunay-Weber Syndrome
(alt: Hemangectatic hypertrophy)

- Organs Involved
  - Blood and/or lymph vessels, face, trunk, limbs, and nervous system rarely

- Diagnostic Characteristics
  - Nevus flammeus (port-wine stain)
  - Venous and lymphatic malformations
  - Hypertrophy of affected limb, gigantism

- Associated Abnormalities
  - AV malformation. High-output heart failure
  - Epilepsy, hypsarrhythmia (rarely)
  - Micropolygyria, hydrocephalus (rarely)

- Differential Diagnosis
  - Sturge-Weber syndrome
  - Epidermal nevus syndrome (linear sebaceum nevus syndrome)

- Genetics
  - Various theories suggested
  - Birth defect associated with translocation at t(q22.3;q13)
  - Associated with VG5Q

- Treatment
  - Surgical
  - Nonsurgical sclerotherapy

- Prognosis
  - High rate of recurrence and complications with therapy

References

Original:
Klippel M, Trenaunay P. Du naevus variqueux osteohypertrophique. Arch Gen Medicine 1900;641–672.
Weber FP. Angioma formation in connection with hypertrophy of limbs and hemi-hypertrophy. Brit Jrnl Dermatology 1907;19:231–235.

Review and Case Reports:
Jacob AG, Driscoll DJ, Shaughnessy WJ, Stanson AW, Clay RP, Gloviczki P. Klippel-Trenaunay syndrome: spectrum and management. Mayo Clin Proc 1998;73(1):28–36.
Howitz P, Howitz J, Gjerris F. A variant of the Klippel-Trenaunay-Weber syndrome with temporal lobe astrocytoma. Acta Paediatr Scand 1979 Jan;68(1):119–121.
Shime H, Araki R, Koide H, Miyaji T, Shioda K. A case of Klippel-Trenaunay-Weber syndrome accompanied by congenital hydrocephalus and micropolygyria. No To Hattatsu 1992 Jul;24(4):353–357.

Kluver-Bucy Syndrome

- Organs Involved
  - Bilateral anterior temporal horns or amygdala
- Diagnostic Characteristics
  - Hyperphagia (pica or bulimia)
  - Hypersexuality
  - Hyperorality
  - Hyperdocility (placidity)
- Associated Abnormalities
  - Visual agnosia (inability to recognize familiar faces, objects, or their use)
  - Hypermetamorphosis (desire to explore everything)
- Etiologies
  - Herpes simplex encephalitis
  - Temporal lobectomy for tumor or epilepsy
  - Stroke, trauma
  - Anoxia, ischemia
  - Dementia, Pick's, or Alzheimer's disease
- Treatment
  - Acyclovir when tied to HSE
  - SSRIs or carbamazepine
- Prognosis
  - Cognitive and behavioral disturbances often severe after HSE
  - Memory loss

References

Original:

Kluver H, Bucy PC. Psychic blindness and other symptoms following bilateral temporal lobectomy in rhesus monkeys. Am J Physiol 1937;119:352–353.

Terzian H, Ore GD. Syndrome of Kluver and Bucy: reproduced in man by bilateral removal of temporal lobes. Neurology 1955 Jun;5(6):373–380.

Review and Case Reports:

Tonsgard JH, Harwicke N, Levine SC. Kluver-Bucy syndrome in children. Pediatr Neurol 1987 May-Jun;3(3):162–165.

Pradhan S, Singh MN, Pandey N. Kluver Bucy syndrome in young children. Clin Neurol Neurosurg 1998 Dec;100(4):254–258.

Janszky J, Fogarasi A, Magalova V, Tuxhom I, Ebner A. Hyperorality in epileptic seizures: periictal incomplete Kluver-Bucy syndrome. Epilepsia 2005 Aug;46(8):1235–1240.

Kile SJ, Ellis WG, Olichney JM, et al. Alzheimer abnormalities of the amygdala with Kluver-Bucy syndrome symptoms: an amygdaloid variant of Alzheimer disease. Arch Neurol 2009 Jan;66(1):125–129.

Kocher-Debre-Semelaigne Syndrome
(alt: Hypothyroid muscular pseudohypertrophy syndrome)

- Organs Involved
  - Muscles, thyroid gland

- Diagnostic Characteristics
  - Generalized muscular hypertrophy ("herculean" appearance)
  - Muscle cramps, pain, and stiffness
  - Congenital hypothyroidism
  - Psychomotor delay

- Differential Diagnosis
  - Duchenne muscular dystrophy
  - Beckwith-Wiederman syndrome (autosomal dominant fetal overgrowth syndrome)

References

Original:
Debre R, Semelaigne G. Syndrome of diffuse hypertrophy in infants causing athletic appearance. Its connection with congenital myxedema. Am J Dis Child 1935;50:1351–1361.

Review and Case Reports:
Shaw C, Shaw P. Kocher-debre-semelaigne syndrome: hypothyroid muscular pseudohypertrophy-a rare report of two cases. Case Report Endocrinol 2012:153143. Epub 2012 Mar 12.
Tashko V, Davachi F, Baboci R, Drishti G, Hoxha P. Kocher-Debre Semelaigne syndrome. Clin Pediatr 1999 Feb;38:113–115.

L

Lambert-Eaton Syndrome – Lowe Syndrome

Lambert-Eaton Syndrome
Lance-Adams Syndrome
Landau-Kleffner Syndrome
Leigh Syndrome
Lennox-Gastaut Syndrome
Lenz Microphthalmia Syndrome (LMS)
Lesch-Nyhan Syndrome
Lewis-Sumner Syndrome
Locked-in Syndrome
Loeys-Dietz Syndrome
Lowe Syndrome

J.G. Millichap, *Neurological Syndromes: A Clinical Guide to Symptoms and Diagnosis*, DOI 10.1007/978-1-4614-7786-0_12,
© Springer Science+Business Media New York 2013

Lambert-Eaton Syndrome

- Organs Involved
  - Neuromuscular junction, lung
- Diagnostic Characteristics
  - Proximal muscle weakness
  - Improved power on repeated hand grip (Lambert's sign)
  - Autonomic symptoms (dry mouth, constipation, orthostatic hypotension)
  - Small cell lung cancer in 60 % (paraneoplastic)
- Associated Abnormalities
  - Autoimmune disease (hypothyroidism, diabetes type 1).
  - Compound motor action potentials (CMAP) small amplitude but normal latency and conduction velocities.
  - CMAP amplitude increases greatly in response to exercise.
- Treatment
  - Chemotherapy and/or radiation for lung neoplasm
  - Pyridostigmine to improve neuromuscular transmission
  - K channel blocker 3,4-diaminopyridine
  - Intravenous immunoglobulin, plasmapheresis for immune suppression

References

Original:

Anderson HJ, Churchill-Davidson HC, Richardson AT. Bronchial neoplasm with myasthenia; prolonged apnoea after administration of succinylcholine. Lancet 1953 Dec;265(6799): 1291–1293.

Lambert EH, Eaton LM, Rooke ED. Defect of neuromuscular conduction associated with malignant neoplasms. Am J Physiol 1956;187:612–613.

Review and Case Reports:

Gutmann L, Crosby TW, Takamori M, Martin JD. The Eaton-Lambert syndrome and autoimmune disorders. Am J Med 1972 Sept;53(3):354–356.

Newsom-Davis J. Lambert-Eaton myasthenic syndrome. Rev Neurol (Paris) 2004 Feb;160(2): 177–180.

Titulaer MJ, Lang B, Verschuuren JJ. Lambert-Eaton myasthenic syndrome: from clinical characteristics to therapeutic strategies. Lancet Neurol 2011 Dec;10(12):1098–1107.

Lance-Adams Syndrome
(alt: Posthypoxic action myoclonus syndrome)

- Organs Involved
  - Brain, cardiopulmonary
- Diagnostic Characteristics
  - Posthypoxic action (or intention) myoclonus developing days or weeks after hypoxic encephalopathy and successful cardiopulmonary resuscitation with regained consciousness
- Associated Abnormalities
  - Asterixis (intermittent lapse of posture [liver flap])
  - Seizures
  - Gait disturbance
- Differential Diagnosis
  - Myoclonic epilepsy
  - Cortical or spinal myoclonus
  - Reflex myoclonus
  - Multifocal myoclonus

References

Original:
Lance JW, Adams RD. The syndrome of intention or action myoclonus as a sequel to hypoxic encephalopathy. Brain. 1963;86(1):111–136.

Review and Case Report:
Lee HL, Lee JK. Lance-Adams syndrome. Ann Rehabil Med 2011 Dec;35(6):939–943.

Landau-Kleffner Syndrome
(alt: Acquired epileptic aphasia syndrome)

- ■ Organs Involved
  - • Cerebral language areas, Broca and Wernicke areas

- ■ Diagnostic Characteristics
  - • Development of aphasia between 3 and 7 years of age
  - • Males predominant 1.7:1
  - • Auditory verbal agnosia, receptive language impaired first, then expressive language impairment
  - • Night seizures and/or epileptiform EEG

- ■ Additional Abnormalities
  - • Behavioral and neuropsychological disorders
  - • ADHD, rage, aggression, anxiety
  - • Short-term memory impairment

- ■ Differential Diagnosis
  - • Autism, PDD
  - • Hearing impairment
  - • Auditory/verbal processing disorder
  - • Learning disability

- ■ Treatment
  - • Anticonvulsants, corticosteroids, ACTH
  - • Speech therapy
  - • Surgery-multiple subpial resection

- ■ Prognosis
  - • Variable, slow, or no recovery
  - • Improved if late onset (after age 6) and speech therapy started early
  - • Seizure remission by adulthood

References

Original:
Landau WM, Kleffner FR. Syndrome of acquired aphasia with convulsive disorder in children. Neurology 1957 Aug;7(8):523–530.

Review and Case Reports:
Sinclair DB, Snyder TJ. Corticosteroids for the treatment of Landau-Kleffner syndrome and continuous spike-wave discharge during sleep. Pediatr Neurol 2005 May;32(5):300–306.
Morrell F, Whisler WW, Smith MC, et al. Landau-Kleffner syndrome. Treatment with subpial intracortical transection. Brain 1995 Dec;118(Pt 6):1529–1546.
Duran MH, Guimaraes CA, Medeiros LL, Guerreiroi MM. Landau-Kleffner syndrome: long-term follow-up. Brain Dev 2009 Jan;31(1):58–63.

Leigh Syndrome
(alt: Subacute necrotizing encephalomyopathy)

- Organs Involved
  - Brainstem and basal ganglia, mitochondrial DNA

- Diagnostic Characteristics
  - Onset first year of life, rarely in adulthood, death within 2 years
  - Presents with vomiting, diarrhea, and dysphagia, failure to thrive
  - Hypotonia and movement disorders (dystonia, tremor, chorea, myoclonus), ataxia
  - Ophthalmoparesis, nystagmus, optic atrophy
  - Episodes of lactic acidosis, hyperventilation, or apnea
  - Hypertrophic cardiomyopathy, impaired respiration

- Associated Abnormalities
  - MRI shows lesions in basal ganglia, cerebellum, brainstem, and brain white matter

- Genetics
  - Mitochondrial DNA mutations in SURF1, MT-ATP6, and other genes cause disruption of cytochrome c oxidase (COX), pyruvate dehydrogenase complex, and ATP synthase, leading to impaired oxidative phosphorylation and cell death, affecting the nervous system, muscles, and heart.

- Treatment
  - High-fat, low-carbohydrate diet, and various vitamins.
  - Vitamin B1 is given for a deficiency in pyruvate dehydrogenase complex.

References

Original:
Leigh DA. Subacute necrotizing encephalomyopathy in an infant. J Neurol, Neurosurg Psychiatry 1951;14:216.

Review and Case Report:
DeVivo DC, Hammond MW, Obert KA, Nelson JS, Pagliara AS. Defective activation of the pyruvate dehydrogenase complex in subacute necrotizing encephalomyopathy (Leigh disease). Ann Neurol 1979 Dec;6(6):483–494.
Macaya A, Munell F, Burke RE, DeVivo DC. Disorders of movement in Leigh syndrome. Neuropediatrics 1993;4(2):60–67.

Lennox-Gastaut Syndrome

- ■ Organs Involved
  - • Cerebral gray matter
- ■ Diagnostic Characteristics
  - • Two or more seizure types including tonic pattern and drop attacks
  - • Slow spike-and-wave EEG pattern, 1.5–2.5 Hz
  - • Slowed psychomotor development
  - • Often preceded by West syndrome
- ■ Treatment
  - • Seizures often resistant
  - • Valproic acid, lamotrigine, topiramate, felbamate, phenytoin, clonazepam
  - • Ketogenic diet

References

Original:
Lennox WG, Davis JP. Clinical correlates of the fast and the slow spike-wave electroencephalogram. Pediatrics 1950 Apr;5(4):626–644.
Gastaut H, Roger J, Soulayrol R, et al. Epileptic encephalopathy of children with diffuse slow spikes and waves (alias "petit mal variant") or Lennox syndrome. Ann Pediatr (Paris) 1966 Aug-Sep;13(8):489–499. [Epilepsia (Amst) 1966;7:139–179].
Niedermeyer E. The Lennox-Gastaut syndrome: a severe type of childhood epilepsy. Deutsch Z. Nervenheilk 1969;195:263–282.

Review and Case Reports:
Camfield PR. Definition and natural history of Lennox-Gastaut syndrome. Epilepsia 2011 Aug;52 Suppl 5:3–9.
VanStraten AF, Ng YT. Update on the management of Lennox-Gastaut syndrome. Pediatr Neurol 2012 Sep;47(3):153–161.

Lenz Microphthalmia Syndrome (LMS)
(alt: Oculofaciocardiodental syndrome)

- Organs Involved
  - Eyes, head, teeth, ears, fingers and toes, skeleton, genitourinary
- Diagnostic Characteristics
  - Microphthalmia, uni- or bilateral/or anophthalmia
  - Coloboma, nystagmus, cataract
  - Low-set ears, anteverted
  - Widely spaced teeth
  - Syndactyly, clinodactyly, duplicated thumbs
  - Microcephaly
  - Kyphoscoliosis, webbed neck
  - Hypospadias, cryptorchidism, renal aplasia
  - Intellectual disability (in 60 % of affected males)
- Genetics
  - Inherited as an X-linked recessive genetic trait, fully expressed in males
  - Mutations of BCOR gene on the X chromosome

References

Review and Case Reports:
Ng D. Lenz microphthalmia syndrome. In: Pagon RA, Bird TD, Dolan CR, Stephens K, Adam MP, editors: GeneReviews, Seattle, WA, University of Washington, Seattle, 1993–2002 Jun 04 [updated 2010 Apr 27].

Lesch-Nyhan Syndrome
(alt: Juvenile gout)

- Organs Involved
  - Joints, blood, kidney, basal ganglia
- Diagnostic Characteristics
  - Neurological dysfunction, hypotonia, dystonia, choreoathetosis, opisthotonus, spasticity
  - Cognitive and compulsive disorders
  - Hyperuricemia and gout
- Associated Abnormalities
  - Kidney stones and damage
  - Self-injurious behavior
- Genetics
  - X-linked recessive inherited disease due to mutations in HPRT1 gene carried by mother and passed to son (one-third de novo cases)
  - Present at birth in baby boys (very rare in girls)
- Treatment
  - Allopurinol to control gout
  - Restraints to prevent self-injury
- Prognosis
  - Poor, death from renal failure in first decade

References

Original:
Lesch M, Nyhan WL. A familial disorder of uric acid metabolism and central nervous system function. Am J Med 1964;36(4):561–570.
Seegmiller JE, Rosenbloom FM, Kelley WN. Enzyme defect associated with a sex-linked human neurological disorder and excessive purine synthesis. Science 1967;155(770):1682–1684.

Review and Case Reports:
Jankovic J, Caskey TC, Stout JT, Butler IJ. Lesch-Nyhan syndrome: a study of motor behavior and cerebrospinal fluid neurotransmitters. Ann Neurol 1988 May;23(5):466–469.
Jinnah HA, Visser JE, Harris JC, et al. Lesch-Nyhan Disease International Study Group. Delineation of the motor disorder of Lesch-Nyhan disease. Brain 2006 May;129(Pt 5): 1201–1217.

Lewis-Sumner Syndrome
(alt: Multifocal acquired demyelinating sensory and motor neuropathy (MADSAM))

- Organs Involved
  - Motor and sensory peripheral nerves

- Diagnostic Characteristics
  - Subacute, painless asymmetric, distal multiple mononeuropathies
  - Distal, asymmetric weakness, mostly upper limbs
  - Multifocal motor conduction blocks
  - Sensory slowing in ulnar and median nerves

- Associated Abnormalities
  - Cranial nerve involvement in 25 % cases
  - Distal limb amyotrophy in 50 %
  - Serum anti-GM1 antibodies absent
  - Chronic progressive course or relapsing remitting

- Differential Diagnosis
  - Multifocal motor neuropathy (with no sensory involvement)
  - Chronic inflammatory demyelinating polyradiculoneuropathy (CIDP)

References

Original:
Lewis RA, Sumner AJ, Brown MJ, Asbury AK. Multifocal demyelinating neuropathy with persistent conduction block. Neurology 1982;32:958

Review and Case Reports:
Viala K, Renie L, Maisonobe T, et al. Follow-up study and response to treatment in 23 patients with Lewis-Sumner syndrome. Brain 2004 Sep;127(Pt 9):2010–2017.

Locked-in Syndrome
(alt: Ventral pontine syndrome)

- Organs Involved
  - Ventral pons damaged (cerebral hemispheres spared)
- Diagnostic Characteristics
  - Quadriplegia
  - Aware and awake but cannot move or communicate verbally
  - Eye movements usually preserved
- Causes
  - Stroke or hemorrhage of basilar artery, affecting ventral pons
  - Central pontine myelinolysis secondary to rapid correction of hyponatremia
  - Traumatic brain injury
  - Medication overdose
- Differential Diagnosis
  - Persistent vegetative state (cerebral hemispheres damaged, brainstem spared)
- Treatment
  - Assistive computer interface technologies, eye tracking
- Prognosis
  - Rare recovery of motor function, 90 % mortality within 4 months of onset
  - Exceptional cases of longer life span or recovery

References

Original:
Plum F, Posner JB. The diagnosis of stupor and coma. Philadelphia, PA: FA Davis, 1966, 197 pp. Idem. Contemp Neurol Ser 1972;10:1–286.

Review and Case Reports:
Bruno MA, Schnakers C, Damas F, et al. Locked-in syndrome in children: report of five cases and review of the literature. Pediatr Neurol 2009 Oct;41(4):237–246.
Nordgren RE, Markesbery WR, Fukuda K, Reeves AG. Seven cases of cerebromedullospinal disconnection: the "locked-in" syndrome. Neurology 1971;21(11):1140–1148.

Loeys-Dietz Syndrome

- ■ Organs Involved
  - • Eyes, palate, arteries, spine, skull, brain, fingers, and toes
- ■ Diagnostic Characteristics
  - • Hypertelorism
  - • Cleft palate, bifid uvula
  - • Aortic dissection and arterial aneurysms with tortuosity
- ■ Associated Abnormalities
  - • Scoliosis
  - • Pectus excavatum
  - • Camptodactyly, long fingers, lax joints
  - • Club foot
  - • Arnold-Chiari malformation
  - • Craniosynostosis
  - • Congenital heart defects
  - • Physical findings similar to Marfan syndrome
- ■ Genetics
  - • Mutations in the genes encoding transforming growth factor beta receptor 1 (TGFBR1) or 2 (TGFBR2) on chromosome 9q22 or 3p22
  - • Autosomal dominant inheritance
- ■ Treatment
  - • Monitor aortic aneurysm formation
  - • NIH sponsored clinical trial of angiotensin II receptor antagonist, losartan to prevent aneurysms in this and Marfan syndromes

References

Original:
Loeys BL, Chen J, Neptune ER, et al. A syndrome of altered cardiovascular, craniofacial, neurocognitive and skeletal development caused by mutations in TGFBR1 or TGFBR2. Nat Genet 2005 Mar;37(3):275–281.
Loeys BL, Schwarze U, Holm T, et al. Aneurysm syndromes caused by mutations in the TGF-beta receptor. N Engl J Med 2006;355(8):788–798.

Review and Case Report:
Rahme RJ, Adel JG, Bendok BR, et al. Association of intracranial aneurysm and Loeys-Dietz syndrome: case illustration, management, and literature review. Neurosurgery 2011 Aug;69(2):E488–492.

Lowe Syndrome
(alt: Oculocerebrorenal syndrome)

- Organs Involved
  - Eyes, central and peripheral nervous systems, kidneys
- Diagnostic Characteristics
  - Congenital cataracts, glaucoma, corneal cheloids
  - Neonatal hypotonia, areflexia
  - Psychomotor retardation
  - Proximal tubular acidosis (Fanconi-type), aminoaciduria, phosphaturia, proteinuria
  - Behavioral problems, seizures, OCD
  - Peripheral neuropathy
- Genetics
  - X-linked recessive, disease in boys only, girls as carriers
  - Mutation of the gene OCRL1 localized at Xq26.1, coding for enzyme phosphatidylinositol phosphatase
- Treatment
  - Correction of tubular acidosis with bicarbonate, phosphate, potassium, water
- Prognosis
  - Life span rarely exceeds 40 years

References

Original:
Lowe CU, Terrey M, MacLachlan EA. Organic-aciduria, decreased renal ammonia production, hydrophthalmos, and mental retardation: a clinical entity. AMA Amer Jrnl Dis Children 1952;83(2):164–184.

Review:
Loi M. Lowe syndrome. Orphanet J Rare Dis 2006 May;18:1–16.

M

Marcus Gunn Syndrome – Muenke Syndrome

Marcus Gunn Syndrome
Marfan Syndrome
Marin Amat Syndrome
Marinesco-Sjogren Syndrome
MASA Syndrome
McLeod Neuroacanthocytosis Syndrome
Meckel-Gruber Syndrome
MECP2 Duplication Syndrome
MEDNIK Syndrome
Meige Syndrome
MELAS Syndrome
Melkersson-Rosenthal Syndrome
MERRF Syndrome
Microphthalmos with Linear Skin Defects Syndrome
Millard-Gubler Syndrome
Miller-Dieker Syndrome
Miller-Fisher Syndrome
Mitochondrial DNA Deletion Syndromes
Mobius Syndrome
Mohr-Tranebjaerg Syndrome
Morvan's Syndrome
Moschcowitz Syndrome
Mowat-Wilson Syndrome
MPV17-Related Hepatocerebral Mitochondrial DNA Depletion Syndrome
Muenke Syndrome

J.G. Millichap, *Neurological Syndromes: A Clinical Guide to Symptoms and Diagnosis*, DOI 10.1007/978-1-4614-7786-0_13,
© Springer Science+Business Media New York 2013

Marcus Gunn Syndrome
(alt: Trigemino-oculomotor synkinesis)

- Organs Involved
  - Muscles supplied by trigeminal and oculomotor nerves
- Diagnostic Characteristics
  - Unilateral congenital ptosis
  - Jaw winking phenomenon – eyelid raised when jaw thrust to opposite side, mouth is opened or infant sucks
  - Cranial nerve synkinesis. Contraction of pterygoid muscles of jaw results in excitation of branch of 3rd Cr nerve that innervates levator palpebrae superioris ipsilaterally
  - Ipsilateral ptosis when mouth is closed
  - Inverse Marcus Gunn phenomenon (Marin Amat syndrome) is rare: ptosis and eye closure when mouth is opened
- Associated Abnormalities
  - Amblyopia in 54 % cases
  - Anisometropia in 26 %
  - Strabismus in 56 %
- Genetics
  - Autosomal dominant with incomplete penetrance
- Treatment
  - Usually unnecessary
  - Reconstructive surgery sometimes indicated

References

Original:
Gunn RM. Congenital ptosis with peculiar associated movements of the affected lid. Trans Ophthal Soc UK 1883;3:283–287.

Review and Case Reports:
Park DH, Choi WS, Yoon SH Treatment of the jaw-winking syndrome. Ann Plast Surg 2008 Apr;60(4):404–409.

Marfan Syndrome

- Organs Involved
  - Connective tissue, limbs, heart, aorta, eye lens, intracranial arteries
- Diagnostic Characteristics
  - Arachnodactyly
  - Long limbs (dolichostenomelia)
  - Coarctation of aorta, valve prolapse
  - Ectopia lentis (upward – superotemporal)
- Associated Abnormalities
  - Scoliosis, back pain, disk disease
  - Dural ectasia encasing the spinal cord
  - Intracranial aneurysm
- Differential Diagnosis
  - Loeys-Dietz syndrome
  - Beals syndrome
  - Ehlers-Danlos syndrome
  - Homocystinuria
  - Shprintzen-Goldberg syndrome
- Genetics
  - Mutations in the FBN1 gene on chromosome 15 that encodes fibrillin-1 protein, essential for integrity of elastic fibers and connective tissue
  - Autosomal-dominant trait, males and females equally affected
- Management
  - Regular cardiology exams to check aortic dilatation. Cardiac surgery
  - Physiotherapy
  - Treat pneumothorax
- History
  - Abraham Lincoln had some of the disease characteristics
  - Paganini and Rachmaninoff may have been affected

References

Original:
Marfan A. Un cas de deformation congenitale des quarter membres, plus pronounces aux extremities caracterisee par l'allongement des os avec un certain degree d'amincissement. Bulletins et memoires de la Societe medicale des hopitaux de Paris. 1896;13(3):220–226.

Review and Case Reports:
Cerullo A, Brayda-Bruno M. Neurological manifestations in Marfan's syndrome. A critical review and presentation of a case. Minerva Med 1992 May;83(5):311–318.
Schievink WI, Parisi JE, Piepgras DG, Michels VV. Intracranial aneurysms in Marfan's syndrome: an autopsy study. Neurosurgery 1997 Oct;41(4):866–870.

Marin Amat Syndrome
(alt: Inverted Marcus Gunn syndrome)

- Organs Involved
  - Muscles supplied by the trigeminal (V) and facial (VII) nerves
- Diagnostic Characteristics
  - Unilateral eye closure or ptosis occurs when mouth is opened or jaw is moved laterally
  - Occurs following recovery from a peripheral facial palsy
  - Associated movement involving facial and masticatory muscles (a synkinesis)

References

Original:
Marin Amat M. Contribucion al studio de la curabiidad de las paralisis oculares de origen traumatico-substitucion funcional de VII por el V par cranial. Archivos de Oftalmologia Hispano-Americanos 1918;18:70–99.

Review and Case Report:
Pavone P, Garozzo R, Trifiletti RR, Parano E. Marin-Amat syndrome: case report and review of the literature. J Child Neurol 1999 Apr;14(4):266–268.

Marinesco-Sjogren Syndrome
(alt: Hereditary oligophrenic cerebello-lental degeneration)

- Organs Involved
  - Cerebellum, eye lens, muscles

- Diagnostic Characteristics
  - Cerebellar ataxia
  - MRI cerebellar vermis atrophy
  - Congenital cataracts
  - Mental retardation
  - Muscle weakness, progressive myopathy

- Associated Abnormalities
  - Small stature
  - Brittle fingernails
  - Sparse hair
  - Speech dysarthria
  - Hypergonadotropic hypogonadism
  - Scoliosis

- Differential Diagnosis
  - Friedreich ataxia
  - Lowe syndrome
  - Other spinocerebellar ataxias

- Genetics
  - Autosomal recessive congenital disorder
  - Mutations of the SIL1 gene in 50 % cases

References

Original:
Marinescu GH, Draganescu S, Vasiliu D. Nouvelle maladie familiale caracterisee par une cataracte congenitale et un arret du development somato-neuro-psychique. L'encephale, Paris, 1931;26:97–109.
Sjogren T. Klinische und vererbungsmedizinische Untersuchungen uber Oligophrenie mit kongenitaler Katarakt. Zeitschrift fur die gesamte Neurologie und Psychiatrie, Berlin. 1935;152:263–292.

Review and Case Report:
Yis U, Cirak S, Hiz S, Cakmakci H, Dirik E. Heterogeneity of Marinesco-Sjogren syndrome: report of two cases. Pediatr Neurol 2011 Dec;45(6):409–411.
Senderek J, Krieger M, Stendel C, et al. Mutations in SIL1 cause Marinesco-Sjogren syndrome, a cerebellar ataxia with cataract and myopathy. Nat Genet 2005 Dec;37(12):1312–1314.

MASA Syndrome
(alt: CRASH syndrome; L1 syndrome)

- Organs Involved
  - Brain, thumbs
- Diagnostic Characteristics
  - **MASA**
  - *M*ental retardation
  - *A*phasia
  - *S*huffling gait
  - *A*dducted thumbs

  - **CRASH**
  - *C*orpus callosum hypoplasia
  - *R*etardation
  - *A*dducted thumbs
  - *S*pastic paraplegia
  - *H*ydrocephalus

- Genetics
  - X-linked recessive
  - Mutations in the L1CAM gene
  - Males affected; female carriers
  - 50 % risk of transfer of affected X chromosome to sons

References

Original:
Bianchine JW, Lewis RC. The MASA syndrome: a new heritable mental retardation syndrome. Clin Genet 1974;5(4):298–306.

Review and Case Reports:
Fransen E, Lemmon V, Van Camp G, Vits L, Coucke P, Williams PJ. CRASH syndrome: clinical spectrum of corpus callosum hypoplasia, retardation, adducted thumbs, spastic paraparesis and hydrocephalus due to mutations in one single gene, L1. Eur J Hum Genet 1995;3(5):273–284.
Yamasaki M, Thompson P, Lemmon V. CRASH syndrome: mutations in L1CAM correlate with severity of the disease. Neuropediatrics 1997 Jun;28(3):175–178.

McLeod Neuroacanthocytosis Syndrome
(Named after the first patient diagnosed, a Harvard dental student)

- Organs Involved
  - Blood cells, muscle, nerves, basal ganglia, heart

- Diagnostic Characteristics
  - Peripheral neuropathy
  - Cardiomyopathy
  - Chorea, tics, lip and tongue biting, dystonia
  - Seizures
  - Late-onset dementia

- Additional Abnormalities
  - Acanthocytes in blood smear
  - Hemolytic anemia
  - Myopathy, elevated creatine kinase
  - MRI T2 signal in putamen, caudate atrophy, gliosis in globus pallidus

- Genetics
  - Recessively inherited mutations in the XK gene on the X chromosome

- Treatment
  - Symptomatic

- Prognosis
  - Slowly progressive

References

Original:
Allen FH Jr, Krabbe SM, Corcoran PA. A new phenotype (McLeod) in the Kell blood-group system. Vox Sang 1961 Sep;6:555–560.

Review and Case Reports:
Danek A, Rubio JP, Rampoldi L, et al. McLeod neuroacanthocytosis: genotype and phenotype. Ann Neurol 2001 Dec;50(6):755–764.

Meckel-Gruber Syndrome
(alt: Meckel's syndrome)

- Organs Involved
  - Brain, kidneys, digits, eyes, palate, heart, face
- Diagnostic Characteristics
  - Occipital encephalocele
  - Polycystic kidneys
  - Polydactyly
  - Microcephaly, anencephaly, cerebellar hypoplasia
  - Microphthalmia, cataracts
- Associated Abnormalities
  - Congenital heart defect
  - Genital anomalies
  - Abnormal facies
  - Polycystic degeneration of kidneys, liver, and pancreas
- Genetics
  - Autosomal recessive inheritance
  - Parental consanguinity in some cases
  - Splice site mutation in the MKS4 gene
  - Diagnosed by fetal DNA analysis and fetal ultrasound in first trimester
  - Diagnosis confirmed at autopsy
- Prognosis
  - Death within days or weeks

References

Original:
Meckel JF. Beschreibung zweier durch sehr ahnliche bildungsabweichungen entstellter geschwister. Deutsches Archiv fur Physiologie 1822;7:99–172.
Gruber GB. Beitrage zur frage "gekoppelter" missbildungen (akrocephalossyndactylie und dysencephalia splancnocystica). Beitr Path Anat 1934;93:459–476.

Review and Case Reports:
Eckmann-Scholz C, Jonat W, Zerres K, Ortiz-Bruchle N. Earliest ultrasound findings and description of splicing mutations in Meckel-Gruber syndrome. Arch Gynecol Obstet 2012 Oct;286(4): 917–921.

MECP2 Duplication Syndrome

- ■ Organs Involved
  - • Brain, muscle, face
- ■ Diagnostic Characteristics
  - • Mental retardation, speech delay
  - • Hypotonia, slow motor development
  - • Progressive spastic paraplegia
  - • Seizures in 50 % affected males
  - • Predisposition to respiratory infections in 75 % males
- ■ Associated Abnormalities
  - • Autism
  - • Gastrointestinal dysfunction
  - • Facial dysmorphism
- ■ Genetics
  - • Duplications of MECP2 are found in all affected males, on chromosome Xq28.
  - • Inherited usually in an X-linked manner, occasionally de novo.
  - • Females who inherit MECP2 duplication are asymptomatic carriers.

References

Reviews and Case Reports:

Echenne B, Roubertie A, Lugtenberg D, Kleefstra T, et al. Neurologic aspects of MECP2 gene duplication in male patients. Pediatr Neurol 2009;41:187–191.

Friez MJ, Jones JR, Clarkson K, et al. Recurrent infections, hypotonia, and mental retardation caused by duplication of MECP2 and adjacent region in Xq28. Pediatrics 2006;118: e1687-1695.

Ramocki MB, Peters SU, Tavyev YJ, et al. Autism and other neuropsychiatric symptoms are prevalent in individuals with MECP2 duplication syndrome. Ann Neurol 2009;66:771–782.

MEDNIK Syndrome

- Organs Involved
  - Liver, copper, hearing, nerves, skin (neurocutaneous)

- Diagnostic Characteristics
  - Mental retardation
  - Deafness
  - Neuropathy
  - Ichthyosis
  - Keratodermia

- Associated Abnormalities
  - Hypocupremia
  - Hypoceruloplasminemia
  - Liver copper accumulation, hepatopathy
  - Intrahepatic cholestasis

- Differential Diagnosis
  - Menkes disease
  - Wilson's disease

- Genetics
  - AP1S1 gene mutations

- Treatment
  - Zinc acetate

References

Original:

Montpetit A, Cote S, Brustein E, et al. Disruption of AP1S1, causing a novel neurocutaneous syndrome, perturbs development of the skin and spinal cord. PLoS Genet 2008 Dec;4(12): e1000296.

Martinelli D, Travaglini L, Drouin CA, et al. MEDNIK syndrome: a novel defect of copper metabolism treatable by zinc acetate therapy. Brain 2013 Mar;136:872-881.

Meige Syndrome
(alt: Brueghel's syndrome, oral facial dystonia)

- Organs Involved
  - Face, jaw
- Diagnostic Characteristics
  - Oromandibular dystonia – chin thrusting, trismus, bruxism, lip pursing, tongue protrusion, dysphagia, dysarthria
  - Blepharospasm symptoms – involuntary increased blinking, squinting, photophobia, uncontrolled eye closure
  - Onset between 30 and 70 years of age; women/men ratio 2:1
- Additional Abnormalities
  - Spasmodic dysphonia, spasmodic torticollis, laryngeal dystonia.
  - Dystonic spasms may be provoked by talking, chewing, or biting.
- Treatment
  - Botox injections
  - Surgery – deep brain stimulation of globus pallidus internus

References

Original:
Meige H. Les convulsions de la face, une forme clinique de convulsion faciale, bilaterale et mediane. Revue Neurologique, Paris. 1910;20:437–443.
Marsden CD. Blepharospasm-oromandibular dystonia syndrome (Brueghel's syndrome). A variant of adult-onset torsion dystonia. Jrnl Neurol, Neurosurgery and Psychiatry, London. 1976;39:1204–1209.

Review and Case Reports:
Reese R, Gruber D, Schoenecker T, et al. Long-term clinical outcome in meige syndrome treated with internal pallidum deep brain stimulation. Mov Disord 2011 Mar;26(4):691–698.
Miyaoka T, Miura S, Seno H, Inagaki T, Horiguchi J. Jaw-opening dystonia (Brueghel's syndrome) associated with cavum septi pellucidi and Verga's ventricle – a case report. Eur J Neurol 2003 Nov;10(6):727–729.

MELAS Syndrome
(alt: Mitochondrial encephalomyopathy, lactic acidosis, and stroke-like episodes)
(Mitochondrial-encephalopathy-lactic acidosis-stroke)

- Organs Involved
  - Mitochondria, brain, hearing
- Diagnostic Characteristics
  - *M*-mitochondrial
  - *E*-encephalopathy
  - *L*-lactic
  - *A*-acidosis
  - *S*-stroke
  - Stroke-like episodes before age 40 years
  - Encephalopathy with seizures and/or dementia
  - Mitochondrial myopathy with lactic acidosis and/or ragged red fibers (RRF) on muscle biopsy
  - Normal early psychomotor development
  - Recurrent headache and vomiting
- Associated Abnormalities
  - Sensorineural hearing loss
  - Generalized tonic-clonic seizures
  - Transient hemiparesis and cortical blindness
  - Impaired mentation
- Genetics
  - Mutations in the mitochondrial DNA (mtDNA) gene MT-TL1 encoding tRNA are causative.
  - MELAS is transmitted by maternal inheritance.
  - The father of a proband is not at risk of having the disease-causing mtDNA mutation.

References

Original:
Hirano M, Ricci E, Koenigsberger MR, et al. Melas: an original case and clinical criteria for diagnosis. Neuromuscul Disord 1992;2(2):125–135.

Review and Case Reports:
Bindoff LA, Engelsen BA. Mitochondrial diseases and epilepsy. Epilepsia 2012 Sep;53 Suppl 4:92–97.

Melkersson-Rosenthal Syndrome
(alt: Rossolimo syndrome)

- ■ Organs Involved
  - • Face, tongue

- ■ Diagnostic Characteristics
  - • Recurrent facial paralysis
  - • Edema of face and lips
  - • Hypertrophy and fissuring of tongue (lingua plicata)
  - • Onset in childhood or adolescence

- ■ Genetics and Etiology
  - • Autosomal-dominant inheritance with variable expressivity
  - • May be symptomatic of Crohn's disease or sarcoidosis

- ■ Treatment
  - • NSAIDs and corticosteroids to reduce swelling
  - • Immunosuppressants and antibiotics
  - • Massage and electrical stimulation

- ■ Prognosis
  - • May become chronic

References

Original:
Melkersson E. En fall av recidiverande facialispares i samband med ett angioneurotiski oedem. Hygiea (Stockholm) 1928;90:737–741.
Rosenthal C. Klinisch-erbbiologischer beitrag zur constitutionspathologie. Gemeinsames auftreten von facialislahmung, angioneurotischem gesichtsodem und lingua plicata in arthritismus-familien. Zeitschrift fur die gesamte Neurologie und Psychiatrie 1931;131:475–450.

Review and Case Reports:
Elias MK, Mateen FJ, Weiler CR. The Melkersson-Rosenthal syndrome: a retrospective study of biopsied cases. J Neurol 2012 Jul 27 [Epub ahead of print]

MERRF Syndrome
(alt: Myoclonic epilepsy associated with ragged red fibers)

- ■ Organs Involved
  - • Multisystem disorder: brain, muscle, eyes
- ■ Diagnostic Characteristics
  - • *M*-Myoclonic
  - • *E*-Epilepsy
  - • *R*-Ragged
  - • *R*-Red
  - • *F*-Fibers
- ■ *Diagnosis* based on: myoclonus, generalized epilepsy, ataxia, and ragged red fibers in muscle biopsy
- ■ Associated Abnormalities
  - • Sensorineural hearing loss
  - • Myopathy
  - • Peripheral neuropathy
  - • Dementia
  - • Short stature
  - • Exercise intolerance
  - • Optic atrophy
  - • Features in <50 % cases: cardiomyopathy, pigmentary retinopathy, pyramidal signs, ophthalmoparesis, multiple lipomas
- ■ Diagnostic Tests
  - • Lactic acid in blood and CSF, CSF protein, EEG, EKG, EMG, MRI (basal ganglia calcification), muscle biopsy, respiratory chain enzymes decreased
- ■ Genetics
  - • MERRF is caused by mutations in mtDNA and is transmitted by maternal inheritance.
  - • Father of a proband is not at risk.
  - • Mother usually has the mtDNA mutation and may or may not have symptoms.

References

Original:
Fukuhara N, et al. 1980; cited in Takeda S, et al. No To Shinkei 1987
Takeda S, Wakabayashi K, Ohama E, et al. An autopsy case of myoclonus epilepsy associated with ragged-red fibers (Fukuhara disease). No To Shinkei 1987 Dec;39(12):1171–1179.

Reviews and Case Reports:
Berkovic SF, Carpenter S, Evans A, et al. Myoclonus epilepsy and ragged-red fibres (MERRF). 1. A Clinical, pathological, biochemical, magnetic resonance spectrographic and positron emission tomographic study. Brain 1989 Oct;112 (Pt5):1231–1260.

Microphthalmos with Linear
Skin Defects Syndrome
(alt: Microphthalmia, dermal aplasia, and scleroderma; MLS syndrome)

- Organs Involved
  - Eye, skin, central nervous system, heart, hearing, genitourinary

- Diagnostic Characteristics
  - Microphthalmia/anophthalmia
  - Linear skin defects on face and neck, heal with age
  - Structural brain defects, agenesis of corpus callosum, microcephaly, hydrocephalus
  - Infantile seizures, intellectual disability, developmental delay
  - Hypertrophic cardiomyopathy

- Associated Abnormalities
  - Short stature
  - Diaphragmatic hernia
  - Hearing loss, preauricular pits
  - Genitourinary malformations
  - Nail dystrophy

- Genetics
  - X-linked inheritance, usually lethal in males
  - Chromosome anomalies involve the Xp22 region
  - HCCS gene mutation

Reference

Morleo M, Franco B. Microphthalmia with linear skin defects syndrome. In: Pagon RA, Bird TD, Dolan CR, Stephens K, Adam MP. Editors. GeneReviews [internet] Seattle (WA): University of Washington, Seattle, 1993–2009 Jun 18 [updated 2011 Aug 18]

Original:
Al-Gazali LI, Mueller RF, Caine A, et al. Two 46, XX, t(X;Y) females with linear skin defects and congenital microphthalmia: a new syndrome at Xp22.3. J Med Genet 1990 Jan;27(1):59–63

Reviews and Case Reports:
Morleo M, Pramparo T, Perone L, et al. Microthalmia with linear skin defects (MLS) syndrome: clinical, cytogenetic, and molecular characterization of 11 cases. Am J Med Genet A 2005 Aug 30;137(2):190–198.

Millard-Gubler Syndrome
(Ventral pontine syndrome)

- Organs Involved
  - Ventral pons, cranial nerves VI and VII
  - Corticospinal tracts
- Diagnostic Characteristics
  - Ipsilateral Cr VI palsy (lateral gaze weakness with diplopia)
  - Ipsilateral Cr VII palsy (peripheral facial weakness)
  - Contralateral hemiplegia (sparing the face) (crossed hemiplegia)
- Causes
  - Basilar artery infarct (paramedian and short circumferential branches) or pontine tumor
  - Unilateral lesion of the ventrocaudal pons
- Differential Diagnosis
  - Other intramedullary brainstem syndromes (Foville, Weber, Claude, Benedikt, Nothnagel, Parinaud, Avellis, Jackson, Wallenberg)

References

Original:
Millard ALJ. Identified the disorder in 1855 (unpublished)
Gubler AM. De l'hemiplegie alterne envisage comme signe de lesion de la protuberance annulaire et comme prevue de la decussation des nerfs faciaux. Gazette hebdomadaire de medicine et de chirurgie, Paris. 1856;3:749–754, 789–792, 811–816.
Foville ALF. Note sur une paralysie peu connue de certains muscles de l'oeil, et sa liaison avec quelques points de l'anatomie de la physiologie de la protuberance annulaire. Gazette hebdomadair de medicine et de chirurgie. 1859;6:146.

Review and Case Reports:
Wolf JK. The Classical Brainstem Syndromes. Springfield, IL, Charles C Thomas, 1971, for translation of original reports (Cited in Adams and Victor's Principles of Neurology, 9th ed, New York, McGraw Hill, 2009, Table 34.3, page 764).

Miller-Dieker Syndrome
(alt: chromosome 17p13.3 deletion syndrome)

- Organs Involved
  - Brain, face
- Diagnostic Characteristics
  - Lissencephaly
  - Craniofacial dysmorphisms
  - Psychomotor delay
  - Multiple abnormalities of brain, heart, kidney, and gastrointestinal tract
- Additional Abnormalities
  - Seizures
  - Failure to thrive
- Genetics
  - Autosomal-dominant inheritance
  - Microdeletion of LIS1 gene on chromosome 17p13
- Prognosis
  - Death in infancy or childhood

References

Original:
Miller JQ. Lissencephaly in two siblings. Neurology 1963;134:841–850.
Dieker H, Edwards RH, ZuRhein G, et al. The lissencephaly syndrome. In: Bergsma D. The Clinical Delineation of Birth Defects: Malformation Syndromes. New York: National Foundation-March of Dimes (pub) II 1969. Pp 53–64.

Reviews and Case Reports:
Nagamani SC, Zhang F, Shchelochkov OA, et al. Microdeletions including YWHAE in the Miller-Dieker syndrome region on chromosome 17p13.3 result in facial dysmorphisms, growth restriction, and cognitive impairment. J Med Genet 2009 Dec;46(12):825–833.

Miller-Fisher Syndrome

- Organs Involved
  - Eye muscles, peripheral nerves
- Diagnostic Characteristics
  - Ophthalmoplegia
  - Ataxia of gait and trunk
  - Areflexia and descending paralysis
  - Variant of acute inflammatory demyelinating polyneuropathy (Guillain Barre syndrome, AIDP)
- Additional Abnormalities
  - An autoimmune disorder, response to foreign antigens (e.g., infection)
  - Anti-GQ1b antibodies, commonly to Campylobacter jejuni
  - CSF protein increased (albumin-cytological dissociation)
  - EMG/NCV: demyelinating neuropathy
  - Response to plasmapheresis is better than IVIg
- Differential Diagnosis
  - Myasthenia gravis
  - Various AIDP subtypes

References

Original:
Fisher CM. An unusual variant of acute idiopathic polyneuritis (syndrome of ophthalmoplegia, ataxia and areflexia). N Engl J Med 1956;255(2):57–65.

Review and Case Reports:
Overell JR, Willison HJ. Recent developments in Miller Fisher syndrome and related disorders. Curr Opin Neurol 2005 Oct;18(5):562–566.
Lee KY. Anti-GQ1b-negative Miller Fisher syndrome after Campylobacter jejuni enteritis. Pediatr Neurol 2012 Sep;47(3):213–215.

Mitochondrial DNA Deletion Syndromes

- Organs Involved
  - Multisystem disorders

- Diagnostic Characteristics

- Three overlapping phenotypes:
  - Kearns-Sayre syndrome (KSS)
  - Pearson syndrome
  - Progressive external ophthalmoplegia (PEO)
  - Rarely, Leigh syndrome

- Kearns-Sayre syndrome:
  - Onset before 20 years of age
  - Pigmentary retinopathy
  - Progressive external ophthalmoplegia (PEO)
  - Cardiac conduction block, CSF protein >100 mg/dl, cerebellar ataxia

- Pearson syndrome:
  - Fatal in infancy, sideroblastic anemia, exocrine pancreas dysfunction (steatorrhea)

- Progressive external ophthalmoplegia:
  - Mitochondrial myopathy
  - Ptosis, ophthalmoplegia
  - Proximal limb weakness

- Genetics
  - Mitochondrial DNA (mtDNA) deletions
  - When inherited, transmitted by maternal inheritance

Reference

Original:
Kearns TP, Sayre GP. Retinitis pigmentosa, external ophthalmoplegia, and complete heart block: unusual syndrome with histologic study in one of two cases. AMA Arch Ophthalmol 1956 Aug;60(2):280–289.

Review and Case Reports:
DiMauro S, Hirano M. Mitochondrial DNA deletion syndromes. In: Pagon RA, Bird TD, Dolan CR, et al. editors. GeneReviews [internet] Seattle (WA) University of Washington, Seattle, 1993-updated May 3 2011.

Mobius Syndrome
(alt: Moebius syndrome)

- Organs Involved
  - Cranial nerves VI and VII, eyes, and face

- Diagnostic Characteristics
  - Facial paralysis, "mask-like" lack of expression
  - Inability to move the eyes from side to side

- Associated Abnormalities
  - Clubbed feet, missing fingers or toes
  - Chest wall abnormalities
  - Strabismus
  - Delayed speech because of lip paralysis
  - Dyspnea and dysphagia
  - Disturbed dentition
  - Corneal erosion due to lack of blinking
  - Increased occurrence of autism

- Cause
  - Prenatal ischemia of brainstem
  - Hypoxia
  - Fetal drug exposure (misoprostol, thalidomide, cocaine)
  - Congenital dysgenesis of cranial nerve nuclei
  - Developmental lesion of lower brainstem (a supranuclear defect), intact facial nuclei
  - Genetic links to 13q12.2 and 1p22. Autosomal dominant in some cases

- Treatment
  - Supportive, in feeding, speech, blinking
  - Surgical "smile surgery"

References

Original:
Mobius PJ. Ueber angeborene doppelseitige Abducens-Facialis-Lahmung. Munchener medizinische Wochenschrift 1888;35:91–94.

Review and Case Reports:
Verzijl HT, Padberg GW, Zwarts MJ. The spectrum of Mobius syndrome: an electrophysiological study. Brain 2005 Jul;128(Pt7):1728–1736.
Gillberg C, Steffenburg S. Autistic behavior in Moebius syndrome. Acta Paediatr Scand 1989 Mar;78(2):314–316.

Mohr-Tranebjaerg Syndrome
(alt: Deafness-Dystonia-Optic Neuronopathy Syndrome)

- Organs Involved
  - Inner ear, brain, eye

- Diagnostic Characteristics
  - Sensorineural hearing loss, profound by age 10 years
  - Dystonia, ataxia
  - Cortical visual impairment, blind in mid-adulthood
  - Changes in personality and aggressive or paranoid behavior
  - Dementia by 40 year of age

- Genetics
  - Mutations in the TIMM8A gene that affect function of mitochondria
  - X-linked recessive progressive disorder

References

Original:
Mohr J, Mageroy K. Sex-linked deafness of a possibly new type. Acta Genet Stat Med 1960;10:54–62.

Review and Case Reports:
Ha AD, Parratt KL, Rendtorff ND, et al. The phenotypic spectrum of dystonia in Mohr-Tranebjaerg syndrome. Mov Disord 2012 Jul;27(8):1034–1040.
Binder J, Hofmann S, Kreisel S, et al. Clinical and molecular findings in a patient with a novel mutation in the deafness-dystonia peptide (DDP1) gene. Brain 2003 Aug;126(Pt 8):1814–1820.

Morvan's Syndrome
(alt: Morvan's fibrillary chorea)

- Organs Involved
  - Muscles, peripheral nerves, brain, autoimmune disorder
- Diagnostic Characteristics
  - Peripheral neuropathy (51 %), pain (62 %), weakness, areflexia
  - Neuropsychiatric features (insomnia 90 %, confusion 66 %, amnesia 56 %, hallucinations 52 %)
  - Dysautonomia (hyperhidrosis 86 %, cardiovascular 48 %, neuropathic pain 62 %)
  - Encephalopathy (generalized tonic-clonic seizures 34 %)
- Associated Abnormalities
  - Voltage-gated potassium channel antibodies in 79 %
  - Autoimmune or paraneoplastic disorder
  - Tumors (41 %), mainly thymomas, associated with high titer CASPR2 antibodies and a poor prognosis
  - LGl1 antibodies associated with serum hyponatremia (25 %)
  - Antibodies binding to multiple brain regions including the hypothalamus and locus coeruleus explains the multifocal phenotypes
  - Similarities to limbic encephalitis (amnesia, seizures, mesial temporal lobe abnormalities). Myokymia, hyperhidrosis, and insomnia favor Morvan syndrome.
  - Myasthenia gravis (31 %)
- Treatment
  - Plasmapheresis
  - Steroids, azathioprine
  - Thymectomy
- Prognosis
  - Variable. Spontaneous remission in some. Death in 9 (31 %) of 29 cases (6 of 12 with tumors, 3 of 17 non-tumor cases)

References

Original:
Morvan AM. De la choree fibrillaire. Gazette hebdomadaire de medicine et de chirurgie, Paris. 1890;27:173–176, 186–189, 200–203.

Reviews and Case Reports:
Liguori R, Vincent L, Clover L, et al. Morvan's syndrome: peripheral and central nervous system and cardiac involvement with antibodies to voltage-gated potassium channels. Brain 2001;124: 2417–2426.
Irani SR, Pettingill P, Kleopa KA, et al. Morvan syndrome: Clinical and serological observations in 29 cases. Ann Neurol 2012 Aug;72(2):241–255.

Moschcowitz Syndrome
(alt: Thrombotic Thrombocytopenic Purpura (TTP))

- Organs Involved
  - Small blood vessels, brain, kidneys, heart
- Diagnostic Characteristics
  - Thrombocytopenia and purpura
  - Microangiopathic hemolytic anemia and jaundice
  - Neurologic symptoms (fluctuating hallucinations, stroke, headaches, posterior reversible encephalopathy syndrome)
  - Kidney failure, hematuria
  - Fever
- Genetics and Etiology
  - Idiopathic and secondary forms and a hereditary form, *Upshaw-Schulman syndrome* (inherited deficiency of ADAMTS13).
  - Idiopathic form of TTP is linked to decrease of enzyme ADAMTS13 and a autoimmune process. ADAMTS13 is responsible for breakdown of Willebrand factor; when breakdown is deficient, coagulation is enhanced, leading to TTP.
  - Secondary TTP may be associated with cancer, pregnancy, HIV-1 infection, or use of certain medications (quinine, immunosuppressants-cyclosporine, interferon).
- Treatment
  - Plasmapheresis
  - Immunosuppressive therapy
  - Prophylactic plasma
- Prognosis
  - Favorable. Most patients recover
  - Abnormal brain MRI does not impact outcome

References

Original:
Moschcowitz E. An acute febrile pleiochromic anemia with hyaline thrombosis of the terminal arterioles and capillaries: an undescribed disease. Proc NY Pathol Soc 1924;24:21–24.

Reviews and Case Reports:
George JN. Thrombotic thrombocytopenic purpura. N Engl J Med 2006;354:1927–1953.
Burrus TM, Wijdicks EF, Rabinstein AA. Brain lesions are most often reversible in acute thrombotic thrombocytopenic purpura. Neurology 2009 Jul;73(1):66–70.

Mowat-Wilson Syndrome
(alt: Hirschsprung Disease-Mental Retardation Syndrome)

- Organs Involved
  - Face, large intestine, corpus callosum, head, eye, genitourinary

- Diagnostic Characteristics
  - Facial: hypertelorism, broad eyebrows, pointed chin, uplifted earlobes
  - Deep set eyes, posteriorly rotated ears
  - Agenesis of corpus callosum
  - Microphthalmia
  - Microcephaly
  - Hirschsprung disease
  - Hypospadias

- Associated Abnormalities
  - Seizures
  - Intellectual disability, speech impairment
  - Growth retardation
  - Behavioral phenotype: oral, repetitive, happy affect, sociable

- Genetics
  - De novo mutations and deletions in the gene ZEB2 (also known as ZFHX1B or SMADIP1) on chromosome 2q22

References

Original:
Mowat DR, Croaker GD, Cass DT, Wilson MJ, et al. Hirschsprung disease, microcephaly, mental retardation, and characteristic facial features: delineation of a new syndrome and identification of a locus at chromosome 2q22-q23. J Med Genet 1998 Aug;35(8):617–623

Review and Case Reports:
Zweier C, Thiel CT, Dufke A, et al. Clinical and mutational spectrum of Mowat-Wilson syndrome. Eur J Med Genet 2005 Apr-Jun;48(2):97–111.
Evans E, Einfeld S, Mowat D, Taffe J, Tonge B, Wilson M. The behavioral phenotype of Mowat-Wilson syndrome. Am J Med Genedt A 2012 Feb;158A(2):358–366.

MPV17-Related Hepatocerebral Mitochondrial DNA Depletion Syndrome

- Organs Involved
  - Liver, brain, central and peripheral nervous systems, mitochondria, parathyroid, kidney, gastrointestine

- Diagnostic Characteristics
  - Infantile-onset jaundice, liver failure, hepatomegaly, cirrhosis
  - Developmental delay
  - Hypotonia, muscle weakness
  - Ataxia
  - Microcephaly
  - Seizures
  - Motor and sensory peripheral neuropathy
  - Leukoencephalopathy
  - Metabolic derangements (lactic acidosis, hypoglycemic crises in infancy)
  - Failure to thrive

- Associated Abnormalities
  - Hypoparathyroidism
  - Renal tubulopathy
  - Gastrointestinal dysmobility
  - Corneal anesthesia

- Genetics
  - Mutations in MPV17 gene which encodes for a mitochondrial membrane protein are causal
  - MtDNA is reduced in liver and muscle tissues
  - Autosomal recessive inheritance

- Prognosis
  - Progressive liver disease leads to death in infancy or early childhood

References

El-Hattab AW, Scaglia F, Craigen WJ, Wong LJC. MPV17-related hepatocerebral mitochondrial DNA depletion syndrome. In: Pagon RA, Bird TD, Dolan CR, Stephens K, Adam MP, editors. GeneReviews [internet]. Seattle (WA): University of Washington, Seattle; 1993–2012 May 17.
Spinazzola A, Santer R, Akman OH, et al. Hepatocerebral form of mitochondrial DNA depletion syndrome: novel MPV17 mutations. Arch Neurol 2008 Aug;65(8):1108–1113.
Merkle AN, Nascene DR, McKinney AM. MR imaging findings in the reticular formation in siblings with MPV17-related mitochondrial depletion syndrome. AJNR Am J Neuroradiol 2012 Mar;33(3):E34–35. Epub 2011 Apr 21.

Muenke Syndrome
(alt: FGFR3-related craniosynostosis)

- Organs Involved
  - Skull, face, toes and fingers, hearing
- Diagnostic Characteristics
  - Unilateral coronal craniosynostosis with anterior plagiocephaly
  - Asymmetry of skull and face
  - Ipsilateral elevation of eyebrow, bossing of forehead
  - Contralateral bulging of frontal bone, depression of eyebrow
- Associated Abnormalities
  - Developmental delay, learning disorder
  - Hypertelorism, ptosis, strabismus
  - Sensorineural hearing loss (mild)
  - Brachydactyly, broad toes and thumbs, clinodactyly
  - Fusion of carpal and tarsal bones on X-ray
  - Epilepsy
- Genetics
  - Pro250Arg mutation in the FGFR3 gene
  - Autosomal-dominant inheritance

References

Original:
Muenke M, Gripp KW, McDonald-McGinn DM, et al. A unique point mutation in the fibroblast growth factor receptor 3 gene (FGFR3) defines a new craniosynostosis syndrome. Am J Hum Genet 1997 Mar;60(3):555–564.

Review and Case Reports:
Agochukwu NB, Doherty ES, Muenke M. Muenke syndrome. In: Pagon RA, Bird TD, Dolan CR, Stephens K, Adam MP, editors. GeneReviews [Internet]. Seattle (WA): University of Washington, Seattle;2006 May 10 [updated 2010 Dec 07].
Doherty ES, Lacbawan F, Hadley DW, Muenke M, et al. Muenke syndrome (FGFR3-related craniosynostosis): expansion of the phenotype and review of the literature. Am J Med Genet A 2007 Dec 15;143A(24):3204–3215.
Agochukwu NB, Solomon BD, Gropman AL, Muenke M. Epilepsy in Muenke syndrome: FGFR3-related craniosynostosis. Pediatr Neurol 2012 Nov;47(5):355–361.

N

Neuroleptic Malignant Syndrome – Nothnagel Syndrome

Neuroleptic Malignant Syndrome
Nijmegen Breakage Syndrome
Noonan Syndrome
Nothnagel Syndrome

J.G. Millichap, *Neurological Syndromes: A Clinical Guide to Symptoms and Diagnosis*, DOI 10.1007/978-1-4614-7786-0_14,
© Springer Science+Business Media New York 2013

Neuroleptic Malignant Syndrome

- ■ Organs Involved
  - • Muscles, autonomic nervous system, brain
- ■ Diagnostic Characteristics
  - • Fever
  - • Encephalopathy (confused or altered consciousness)
  - • *V*itals unstable (autonomic [blood pressure] instability)
  - • *E*levated enzymes (CPK) and white blood cells
  - • *R*igidity of muscles, cramps, and tremors
- ■ Associated Abnormalities
  - • Neuroleptic drug use (haloperidol, chlorpromazine) also, levodopa withdrawal
  - • Sudden reduction in dopamine activity
  - • Dementia patients at increased risk
  - • Low serum iron
- ■ Differential Diagnosis
  - • Encephalitis, toxic encephalopathy
  - • Status epilepticus
  - • Heat stroke, malignant hyperthermia
  - • Serotonin syndrome (excess serotonergic activity)
- ■ Treatment
  - • Stop neuroleptic drugs and treat hyperthermia aggressively
  - • Dantrolene most effective, bromocriptine also recommended
  - • Benzodiazepines to control agitation but may increase risk of NMS
  - • Intravenous hydration as necessary
- ■ Prognosis
  - • Mortality rate <10 %

References

Original:
Delay J, Pichot P, Lemperier MT, Ellisalde B, Peigne F. Un neuroleptique majeur non phenothi-azineque et non reserpinique, l'halidol, dans le traitement des psychoses. Ann Med Psychol (Paris) 1960;118:145–152.

Review and Case Reports:
Nielsen RE, Wallenstein Jensen SO, Nielsen J. Neuroleptic malignant syndrome-an 11-year longi-tudinal case–control study. Can J Psychiatry 2012 Aug;57(8):512–518.
Perry PJ, Wilborn CA. Serotonin syndrome vs neuroleptic malignant syndrome: a contrast of causes, diagnoses, and management. Ann Clin Psychiatry 2012 May;24(2):155–162.

Nijmegen Breakage Syndrome
(alt: Berlin Breakage Syndrome; Seemanova syndrome)

- Organs Involved
  - Skull, face, lung, brain

- Diagnostic Characteristics
  - Microcephaly
  - Growth retardation, short stature
  - Facial features: sloping forehead, receding mandible, prominent nose, large ears, upward slant of palpebral fissures
  - Recurrent sinopulmonary infections
  - Malignancies (B-cell lymphoma) before age 15 years
  - Intellectual disability by age 10 years

- Genetics
  - Mutations in NBN gene. Autosomal recessive inheritance
  - Inversions and translocations involving chromosomes 7 and 14
  - Most cases have West Slavic origin, chiefly Poland

References

Original:

Weemaes CM, Hustinx TW, Scheres JM, van Munstr PJ, Bakkeren JA, Taalman RD. A new chromosomal instability disorder: the Nijmegen breakage syndrome. Acta Paediatr Scand 1981;70(4):557–564.

Reviews and Case Reports:

Concannon P, Gatti R. In: Pagon RA, Bird TD, Dolan CR, et al., editors. GeneReviews [internet] Seattle(WA): University of Washington, Seattle, 1993- [last update Mar 1, 2011]

International Nijmegen Breakage Syndrome Study Group. Nijmegen breakage syndrome. Arch Dis Child 2000 May;82(5):400–406.

Chrzanowska KH, Gregorek H, Dembowska-Baginska B, Kalina MA, Digweed M. Nijmegen breakage syndrome (NBS). Orphanet J Rare Dis 2012 Feb 28;7:13.

Noonan Syndrome

- ■ Organs Involved
  - • Heart, face, neck, brain, blood
- ■ Diagnostic Characteristics
  - • Pulmonary valvular stenosis and other congenital cardiac defects
  - • Short stature, psychomotor delay, and learning disabilities
  - • Hypertelorism, epicanthal folds, webbed neck, low-set ears and hairline
  - • Deep philtrum, micrognathia, dysarthria, speech delay
  - • Cryptorchidism
- ■ Associated Abnormalities
  - • Arnold-Chiari type 1, moyamoya
  - • Macrocephaly
  - • Incoordination
  - • Scoliosis, pectus excavatum
  - • Blood clotting disorders
- ■ Genetics
  - • Autosomal dominant inheritance
  - • No chromosomal defect, both sexes affected
  - • Mutations in the Ras/mitogen-activated protein kinase in ~70 % cases
- ■ Differential Diagnosis
  - • Turner syndrome
  - • Fetal alcohol syndrome
  - • Leopard syndrome
  - • Cardiofaciocutaneous syndrome

References

Original:
Noonan JA. Hypertelorism with Turner phenotype. A new syndrome with associated congenital heart disease. Am J Dis Child 1968 Oct;116(4):373–380.
Noonan JA. Noonan syndrome revisited. J Pediatr 1999 Dec;135(6):667–668.

Review and Case Reports:
Schon F, Bowler J, Baraitser M. Cerebral arteriovenous malformation in Noonan's syndrome. Postgrad Med J 1992 Jan;68(795):37–40.
Ganesan V, Kirkham FJ. Noonan syndrome and moyamoya. Pediatr Neurol 1997 Apr;16(3): 256–258.
Van der Burgt I, Thoonen G, Roosenboom N et al. Patterns of cognitive functioning in school-aged children with Noonan syndrome associated with variability in phenotypic expression. J Pediatr 1999 Dec;135(6):707–713.

Nothnagel Syndrome
(alt: Dorsal midbrain syndrome)

- Organs Involved
  - Oculomotor nucleus, superior cerebellar peduncle of midbrain
- Diagnostic Characteristics
  - Ipsilateral oculomotor palsy and gaze paralysis
  - Contralateral cerebellar ataxia
  - Tumor impacting superior cerebellar peduncle

References

Original:
Nothnagel CWH. Topische diagnostik der gehirnkrankheiten: Eine klinische studie. Berlin, A Hirschwald, 1879, p 220.

Review and Case Reports:
Schmidt D. Classical brain stem syndrome. Definitions and history. Ophthalmologe 2000 Jun;97(6):411–417.
Derakhshan I, Sabouri-Deylami M, Kaufman B. Bilateral Nothnagel syndrome. Clinical and roentgenological observations. Stroke 1980 Mar-Apr;11(2):177–179.
Liu GT, Crenner CW, Logigian EL, Charness ME, Samuels MA. Midbrain syndromes of Benedikt, Claude, and Nothnagel: setting the record straight. Neurology 1992 Sep;42(9):1820–1822.

O

OHAHA Syndrome – Osler-Weber-Rendu Syndrome

OHAHA Syndrome
Ohtahara Syndrome
Opitz Syndrome
Opsoclonus Myoclonus Syndrome
Oral-Facial-Digital Syndrome Type 1
Osler-Weber-Rendu Syndrome

J.G. Millichap, *Neurological Syndromes: A Clinical Guide to Symptoms and Diagnosis*, DOI 10.1007/978-1-4614-7786-0_15,
© Springer Science+Business Media New York 2013

OHAHA Syndrome
(alt: Infantile onset spinocerebellar ataxia (IOSCA))

- Organs Involved
  - Central and peripheral nervous system, eyes, inner ear, cerebellum

- Diagnostic Characteristics
  - *O*-Ophthalmoplegia
  - *H*-Hypotonia
  - *A*-Ataxia
  - *H*-Hypoacusis
  - *A*-Athetosis

- Associated Abnormalities
  - Optic atrophy
  - Seizures
  - Axonal neuropathy

- Differential Diagnosis
  - Kearns-Sayre, other mitochondrial disorders, MELAS, MERRF

References

Original:
Kallio AK, Jauhiainen T. A new syndrome of ophthalmoplegia, hypoacusis, ataxia, hypotonia, and athetosis (OHAHA). Adv Audiol 1985;3:84–90.

Review and Case Reports:
Santavuori P, Vihavainen J. Personal communication on OHAHA syndrome to McKusick VA. Mendelian Inheritance in Man; A Catalog of Human Genes and Genetic Disorders, 12th ed. Baltimore: The Johns Hopkins University Press, 1998.
Hakonen AH, Goffart S, Marjavaara S, et al. Infantile-onset spinocerebellar ataxia and mitochondrial recessive ataxia syndrome are associated with neuronal complex 1 defect and mtDNA. Hum Mol Genet 2008 Dec 1;17(23):3822–3835.

Ohtahara Syndrome
(alt: Early infantile epileptic encephalopathy with burst- suppression, EIEE)

- Organs Involved
  - Brain

- Diagnostic Characteristics
  - Refractory tonic seizures 10–300 times daily; less often partial seizures
  - Seizure onset in first 10 days to 3 weeks of life
  - May evolve into West syndrome and Lennox-Gastaut syndrome
  - Burst-suppression pattern on EEG
  - Progressive mental and physical retardation

- Differential Diagnosis
  - Early myoclonic encephalopathy (no unique evolution)
  - West syndrome
  - Late infantile epileptic encephalopathy
  - Lennox-Gastaut syndrome

- Cause
  - No single cause identified. Various clinical and EEG features of epileptic encephalopathies are probably age and brain maturation dependent.
  - Brain atrophy or malformation.
  - Metabolic.
  - Genetic mutations.

- Genetics
  - Several genes associated including ARX, CDKL5, KCNQ2

- Treatment
  - Steroids, ACTH, and anticonvulsant drugs of limited effect

- Prognosis
  - Intractable seizures and severe mental retardation

References

Original:
Ohtahara S, Ishida T, Oka E, et al. On the specific age dependent epileptic syndrome: the early-infantile epileptic encephalopathy with suppression-burst. No to Hattatsu 1976;8:270–279.

Review and Case Reports:
Ohtahara S, Yamatogi Y. Epileptic encephalopathies in early infancy with suppression-burst. J Clin Neurophysiol 2003 Nov-Dec;20(6):398–407.
Nordli DR Jr. Epileptic encephalopathies in infants and children. J Clin Neurophysiol 2012 Oct;29(5):420–424.
Beal JC, Cherian K, Moshe SL. Early-onset epileptic encephalopathies: Ohtahara syndrome and early myoclonic encephalopathy. Pediatr Neurol 2012 Nov;47(5):317–323.

Opitz Syndrome
(alt: X-linked Opitz G/BBB syndrome; XLOS)

- Organs Involved
  - Face, larynx, genitourinary, heart, brain
- Diagnostic Characteristics
  - Hypertelorism, prominent forehead, cleft lip and palate
  - Hypospadias, laryngotracheoesophageal defects
  - Midline brain defects (Dandy-Walker, corpus callosum and cerebellar vermis agenesis)
- Genetics
  - Mutations in gene MID1
  - X-linked or autosomal dominant inheritance

References

Original:
Opitz JM, Summitt RL, Smith DW. The BBB syndrome familial telecanthus with associated congenital anomalies. Birth Defects. Original Article Series. 1969b;2(V):86–94.

Review and Case Reports:
Meroni G. X-linked Opitz G/BBB syndrome. In: Pagon RA, Bird TD, Dolan CR, et al., editors. Gene Reviews [Internet]. Seattle (WA): University of Washington, Seattle, 2004 Dec 17 [updated 2011 Jul 28].
Hu CH, Liu YF, Yu JS, et al. A MID1 gene mutation in a patient with Opitz G/BBB syndrome that altered the 3D structure of SPRY domain. Am J Med Genet A 2012 Apr;158A(4):726–731.
De Falco F, Cainarca S, Andolfi G, et al. X-linked Opitz syndrome: novel mutations in the MID1 gene and redefinition of the clinical spectrum. Am J Med Gernet A 2003 Jul 15;120A(2): 222–228.

Opsoclonus Myoclonus Syndrome
(alt: Dancing eyes syndrome; Kinsbourne syndrome)

- Organs Involved
  - Eyes, trunk, limbs, diaphragm, larynx, pharynx

- Diagnostic Characteristics
  - Random, high-amplitude, arrhythmic, multidirectional, involuntary conjugate eye movements
  - Focal or diffuse myoclonus, involving trunk, limbs, diaphragm, larynx, pharynx
  - Aphasia, mutism
  - Lethargy, sleep disorder
  - May be self-limiting when associated with viral encephalitis
  - When occurring with neuroblastoma in children, associated with anti-Hu (ANNA-!) antibodies
  - In adults, occurs with small cell lung carcinoma or breast carcinoma and associated with anti-Hu (ANNA-1) or anti-Ri (ANNA-2) antibodies

- Treatment and Prognosis
  - In children, surgery for removal of neuroblastoma and ACTH or corticosteroids. Good response usual but may have long-term developmental and cognitive problems
  - In adults, worse prognosis for paraneoplastic syndrome cases

References

Original:
Kinsbourne M. Myoclonic encephalopathy of infants. J Neurol Neurosurg Psychiatr 1962 Aug;25(3):271–276.

Review and Case Reports:
Koh PS, Raffernsperger JG, Berry S, Larsen MB, et al. Long-term outcome in children with opsoclonus-myoclonus and ataxia and coincident neuroblastoma. J Pediatr 1994 Nov;125(5Pt 1):712–716.

Oral-Facial-Digital Syndrome Type 1
(alt: Papillon-League and Psaume syndrome)

- Organs Involved
  - Tongue, teeth, face, hands, brain, kidney
- Diagnostic Characteristics
  - Bifid lobed tongue with nodules, ankyloglossia, short frenulum
  - Cleft palate, missing teeth
  - Hypertelorism, cleft lip, micrognathia
  - Brachydactyly, syndactyly, polydactyly
  - Duplicated great toe
  - Intracerebral cysts, agenesis of corpus callosum, cerebellar agenesis
  - Intellectual disability
  - Renal cysts, polycystic kidney disease
- Genetics
  - Inherited as X-linked dominant manner.
  - Mutation in OFD1 gene located on the X chromosome
  - Related to the ciliopathies (e.g., Bardet-Biedl syndrome, polycystic kidney disease, Meckel-Gruber syndrome)

References

Badano JL, Mitsuma N, Beales PL, Katsanis N. The ciliopathies: an emerging class of human genetic disorders. Annu Rev Genomics Hum Genet 2006;7:125–148,

Towfighi J, Berlin CM Jr, Ladda RL, Frauenhoffer EE, Lehman RA. Neuropathology of oral-facial-digital syndromes. Arch Pathol Lab Med 1985 Jul;109(7):642–646.

Odent S, Le Marec B, Toutain A, et al. Central nervous system malformations and early end-stage renal disease in oro-facio-digital syndrome type 1: a review. Am J Med Genet 1998 Feb 3;75(4):389–394.

Holub M, Potocki L, Bodamer OA. Central nervous systems malformations in oral-facial-digital syndrome, type 1. Am J Med Genet A 2005 Jul 15;136(2):218.

O   OHAHA Syndrome – Osler-Weber-Rendu Syndrome

Osler-Weber-Rendu Syndrome
(alt: Hereditary hemorrhagic telangiectasia (HHT))

- Organs Involved
  - Blood vessels in skin, mucous membranes, lungs, liver, brain
- Diagnostic Characteristics (Curacao criteria)
  - Recurrent epistaxis
  - Multiple telangiectasias
  - Arteriovenous malformations in brain (10 %), lungs (50 %), liver (30–70 %)
  - First-degree family member with HHT
- Genetics
  - Sequence analysis testing indicated in "possible" cases
  - ENG, ACVRL1, and MADH4 mutation tests available
  - HHT highest incidence in Curacao, Netherlands Antilles
- Prognosis
  - Normal life span usual
  - Frequent nosebleeds most troublesome symptom

References

Original:
Osler W. On a family form of recurring epistaxis, associated with multiple telangiectases of the skin and mucous membranes. Bull Johns Hopkins Hosp 1901;12:333–337.
Weber FP. Multiple hereditary developmental angiomata (telangiectases) of the skin and mucous membranes associated with recurring haemorrhages. Lancet 1907;2(4377):160–162.
Rendu HJJ. Epistaxis repetees chez un sujet porteur de petits angiomes cutanes et muqueux. Gaz Hop 1896;1322–1323.

Review and Case Reports:
Faughnan ME, Palda VA, Garcia-Tsao G, et al. International guidelines for the diagnosis and management of hereditary haemorrhagic telangiectasia. J Med Genet 2011;48(2):73–87.

P

Pallister-Hall Syndrome – Proteus Syndrome

Pallister-Hall Syndrome
Panayiotopoulos Syndrome
Paraneoplastic Syndrome
Parinaud Syndrome
Parry-Romberg Syndrome
Parsonage-Turner Syndrome
Patau Trisomy 13 Syndrome
PEHO Syndrome
Pena-Shokeir Syndrome
Pendred Syndrome/DFNB4
Perry Syndrome
Pfeiffer Syndrome Type 2
PHACES Syndrome
Phelan-McDermid Syndrome
Pitt-Hopkins Syndrome
POEMS Syndrome
Poland Syndrome
Prader-Willi Syndrome
Proteus Syndrome

J.G. Millichap, *Neurological Syndromes: A Clinical Guide to Symptoms and Diagnosis*, DOI 10.1007/978-1-4614-7786-0_16,
© Springer Science+Business Media New York 2013

Pallister-Hall Syndrome

- Organs Involved
  - Hypothalamus, fingers, epiglottis, kidney

- Diagnostic Characteristics
  - Hypothalamic hamartoma in floor of third ventricle
  - Postaxial (ulnar) polydactyly
  - Bifid epiglottis

- Associated Abnormalities
  - Renal cysts or hypoplasia
  - Imperforate anus

- Genetics
  - Mutations of gene GLI3

References

Original:

Marcuse PM, et al. Hamartoma of the hypothalamus: Report of two cases with associated developmental defects. J Pediatr, St Louis 1953;43:301–306.

Hall JG, Pallister PD, Clarren SK, et al. Congenital hypothalamic hamartoblastoma, hypopituitarism, imperforate anus, and postaxial polydactyly – a new syndrome? Part I. Clinical, causal, and pathogenic considerations. Am J Med Genet, New York 1980;7:47–74.

Clarren SK, et al. Congenital hypothalamic hamartoblastoma, hypopituitarism, imperforate anus, and postaxial polydactyly – a new syndrome? II. Neuropathological considerations. Am J Med Genet, New York 1980;7:75–83.

Review and Case Reports:

Boudreau EA, Liow K, Frattali CM, et al. Hypothalamic hamartomas and seizures: distinct natural history of isolated and Pallister-Hall syndrome. Epilepsia 2005 Jan;46(1):42–47.

Panayiotopoulos Syndrome

- Diagnostic Characteristics
  - Early-onset benign childhood seizures with occipital spikes, now referred to as "Panayiotopoulos syndrome (PS)" or "Panayiotopoulos type of benign childhood occipital epilepsy."
  - Infrequent partial seizures or partial status of autonomic and behavioral pattern, including ictal vomiting, tonic deviation of eyes, and impaired consciousness, followed by generalized tonic-clonic seizures.
  - Peak age of onset 5 years (late onset or Gastaut type of childhood epilepsy with occipital paroxysms (CEOP) has onset of 8–9 years).
  - EEG occipital spikes disappear with eye opening and reappear with eye closure.
- Differential Diagnosis
  - Myoclonic, absence, and photosensitive epilepsies (may have EEG occipital spikes similar to PS)
  - Epilepsy with occipital calcifications
  - Sturge-Weber syndrome
  - Infantile neuronal ceroid lipofuscinosis
  - Migraine
  - Cyclic vomiting
- Prognosis
  - Excellent, resolution within several years of onset.
  - Occasionally seizures persist in to adult life.

References

Original:
Panayiotopoulos CP. Benign childhood epilepsy with occipital paroxysms: a 15-year prospective study. Ann Neurol 1989;26:51–56.
Panayiotopoulos CP. Benign nocturnal childhood occipital epilepsy: a new syndrome with nocturnal seizures, tonic deviation of the eyes, and vomiting. J Child Neurol 1989;4:43–49.

Review and Case Reports:
Mosely B, Bateman L, Millichap JJ, Wirrell E, Panayiotopoulos CP. Autonomic epileptic seizures, autonomic effects of seizures and SUDEP. Epilepsy Behav 2012 Oct 22 [Epub ahead of print]
Specchio N, Trivisano M, Claps D, Battagli D, Fusco L, Vigevano F. Documentation of autonomic seizures and autonomic status epilepticus with ictal EEG in Panayiotopoulos syndrome. Epilepsy Behav Nov;19(3):383–393.
Ahmed Sharoqi I A, Parker A, Agathonikou A. Early onset benign childhood occipital seizures (Panayiotopoulos' syndrome). Epilepsia 1997;38 Suppl 3:223.

Paraneoplastic Syndrome

- Organs Involved
  - Nervous, muscular, endocrine, mucocutaneous, hematological systems
- Diagnostic Characteristics
  - Cancers associated are breast, ovarian, lung, or lymphatic system.
  - Symptoms include ataxia, dizziness, nystagmus, dysphagia, hypotonia, incoordination, dysarthria, memory loss, visual disturbance, sleep problems, dementia, seizures, sensory loss.
- Neurologic Syndrome and Associated Cancer (in Parenthesis)
  - Lambert-Eaton myasthenic syndrome (LEMS) (small-cell lung cancer)
  - Cerebellar degeneration (lung, ovarian, or breast)
  - Limbic encephalitis (small-cell lung)
  - Opsoclonus myoclonus (neuroblastoma in children, breast, ovarian, lung)
  - Anti-NMDA receptor encephalitis (teratoma)
  - Polymyositis (lymphoma, lung, bladder)
  - Sensorimotor polyneuropathy (all types of cancer)
- Treatment
  - Chemotherapy, radiation, and surgery to eliminate cancer
  - Symptomatic, steroids, ACTH

References

Reviews:

Darnell RB, Posner JB. Paraneoplastic Syndromes. Oxford University Press, 2011;pp 496

Inuzuka T. Paraneoplastic neurological syndrome—definition and history. Brain Nerv 2010 Apr;62(4):301–308.

Darnell RB, DeAngelis LM. Regression of small-cell lung carcinoma in patients with paraneoplastic neuronal antibodies. Lancet 1993;341(8836):21–22.

Koh PS, Raffensperger JG, Berry S, Larsen MB, et al. Long-term outcome in children with opsoclonus-myoclonus and ataxia and coincident neuroblastoma. J Pediatr 1994 Nov;125(5 Pt1):712–716.

Klaas JP, Ahlskog JE, Pittock SJ, et al. Adult-onset opsoclonus-myoclonus syndrome. Arch Neurol 2012 Sep 17:1–10 [Epub ahead of print]

Parinaud Syndrome
(alt: Dorsal midbrain syndrome)

- Organs Involved
  - Eye and upper brainstem, pretectum, superior colliculi

- Diagnostic Characteristics
  - Dorsal midbrain lesion
  - Supranuclear upgaze palsy
  - Eyelid retraction (Collier's sign)
  - Convergence retraction nystagmus (on attempted upward gaze)

- Associated Abnormalities
  - Pseudo-Argyll Robertson pupils
  - Bilateral papilledema
  - Pinealoma
  - Multiple sclerosis
  - Stroke of upper brainstem, aneurysm
  - Metabolic disorders (kernicterus, Wilson's disease, Niemann-Pick)

- Treatment and Prognosis
  - Ventriculoperitoneal shunt followed by slow resolution over 3–6 months
  - Eye muscle surgery for inferior rectus recessions

References

Original:
Parinaud H. Paralysie des mouvements associes des yeux. Archives de neurologie, Paris. 1883;5:145–172.

Review and Case Reports:
Yiu G, Lessell S. Dorsal midbrain syndrome from a ring-enhancing lesion. Semin Ophthalmol 2012 May-Jul;27(3–4):65–68.
Gregory ME, Rahman MQ, Cleary M, Weir CR. Dorsal midbrain syndrome with loss of motor fusion: a rare association. Strabismus 2011 Mar;19(1):17–20.
Goldenberg-Cohen N, Haber J, Ron Y, et al. Long-term ophthalmological follow-up of children with Parinaud syndrome. Ophthalmic Surg Lasers Imaging 2010 Jul-Aug;41(4):467=471.

Parry-Romberg Syndrome
(alt: Romberg's disease)

- Organs Involved
  - Face, tongue, gingiva, soft palate, cartilage, trigeminal nerve
- Diagnostic Characteristics
  - Facial hemiatrophy; bilateral in 5–10 % cases
  - Hemiatrophy of tongue, soft palate, cartilage of nose, and larynx
  - Localized scleroderma with frontal alopecia (coup de sabre)
  - Onset in childhood, females more than males
- Associated Abnormalities
  - Neurological: trigeminal neuralgia, migraine, seizures
  - Ocular: Horner's syndrome, ophthalmoplegia
- Etiology
  - Autoimmune disease and other causes
  - Sometimes familial; autosomal dominant inheritance suggested
- Treatment
  - Immunosuppressive drugs sometimes helpful
  - Reconstructive surgery

References

Original:
Parry CH. Facial hemiatrophy. In Parry CH: Collections from the unpublished medical writings of the late Caleb Hillier Parry, Vol I, London, Underwood, Fleet Street, 1825. Pp 478–480.
Von Romberg MH. Trophoneurosen. In Romberg: Klinische Ergebnisse. Berlin, Forstner, 1846, pp 75–81.

Reviews and Case Reports:
Viana M, Glastonbury CM, Sprenger T, Goadsby PJ. Trigeminal neuropathic pain in a patient with progressive facial hemiatrophy (parry-romberg syndrome). Arch Neurol 2011 Jul;68(7): 938–943.
Rogers BO. Progressive facial hemiatrophy: Romberg's disease: a review of 772 cases. Proceedings of the 3rd International Conference on Plastic Surgery. Excerpta Medica. International Congress Series, 1963;66:681–686.

Parsonage-Turner Syndrome
(alt: Parsonage-Aldren-Turner syndrome, neuralgic amyotrophy, acute brachial neuropathy)

- Organs Involved
  - Brachial plexus, usually suprascapular and axillary nerves and corresponding supraspinatus, infraspinatus, and deltoid muscles

- Diagnostic Characteristics
  - Acute severe shoulder or arm pain followed by weakness and numbness
  - Muscle atrophy
  - Usually idiopathic; sometimes associated with viral infection
  - Recovery slow but usually complete in 18–24 months

- Differential Diagnosis
  - Hereditary neuralgic amyotrophy

- Treatment
  - Usually supportive
  - Some reports of more rapid recovery following steroids and IV immunoglobulin

References

Original:
Parsonage MJ, Turner JW. Neuralgic amyotrophy: the shoulder-girdle syndrome. Lancet 1948 June; Lancet 1(6513):973–978.

Review and Case Reports:
Hussey AJ, O'Brien CP, Regan PJ. Parsonage-Turner syndrome-case report and literature review. Hand (NY) 2007 Dec;2(4):218–221.
Tjoumakaris FP, Anakwenze OA, Kancheria V, Pulos N. Neuralgic amyotrophy (Parsonage-Turner syndrome). J Am Acad Orthop Surg 2012 Jul;20(7):443–449.

Patau Trisomy 13 Syndrome

- Organs Involved
  - Brain, spine, musculoskeletal, cutaneous, urogenital, heart
- Diagnostic Characteristics
  - Microcephaly, holoprosencephaly
  - Microphthalmos
  - Meningomyelocele
  - Polydactyly, overlapping of fingers, rocker bottom feet
- Associated Abnormalities
  - Cleft palate
  - Heart defects
  - Genitalia and kidney defects
- Genetics
  - Trisomy 13 or partial trisomy 13 in most cases
  - Usually random but may be inherited
- Prognosis
  - >80 % die within first year of life

References

Original:
Patau K, Smith DW, Therman E, Inhorn SL, Wagner HP. Multiple congenital anomaly caused by an extra autosome. Lancet 1960;1(7128):790–793.

Review and Case Reports:
Janvier A, Farlow B, Wilfond BS. The experience of families with children with trisomy 13 and 18 in social networks. Pediatrics 2012 Aug;130(2):293–298.

PEHO Syndrome
(alt: Progressive encephalopathy, hypsarrhythmia, and optic atrophy syndrome)
(Infantile cerebello-optic atrophy syndrome)

- **Organs Involved**
  - Visual pathways, cerebellum, cerebrum, lymphatics

- **Diagnostic Characteristics**
  - *P*-Progressive
  - *E*-Encephalopathy
  - *H*-Hypsarryhthmia
  - *O*-Optic atrophy

- **Associated Abnormalities**
  - Seizures
  - Cerebellar hypoplasia or aplasia
  - Microcephaly, cerebral cortex atrophy
  - Mental retardation
  - Scoliosis
  - Hypotonia
  - Lymphedema

- **Genetics**
  - Autosomal recessive likely
  - Mostly Finnish families

References

Original:
Salonen R, Somer M, Haltia M, Lorentz M, Norio R. Progressive encephalopathy with edema, hypsarrhythmia, and optic atrophy (PEHO syndrome). Clin Genet 1991;39:287–293.

Review and Case Reports:
Somer M. Diagnostic criteria and genetics of the PEHO syndrome. J Med Genet 1993 Nov;30(11): 932–936.
Chitty LS, Robb S, Berry C, Silver D, Baraitser M. PEHO or PEHO-like syndrome? Clin Dysmorph 1996;5:143–152.

Pena-Shokeir Syndrome
(alt: Fetal akinesia deformation sequence; arthrogryposis multiplex congenita with pulmonary hypoplasia)

- Organs Involved
  - Joints and limbs, craniofacial, lungs, spinal cord, brain
- Diagnostic Characteristics
  - Lack of fetal movement (fetal akinesia deformation sequence)
  - Joint contractures (arthrogryposis)
  - Craniofacial abnormalities (hypertelorism, prominent nasal bridge)
  - Pulmonary hypoplasia
- Associated Abnormalities
  - Microcephaly
  - Diaphragmatic hernia
  - Micrognathia
- Genetics
  - Autosomal recessive most common transmission
  - Many (~20) familial subtypes; mostly sporadic
- Differential Diagnosis
  - Trisomy 18
  - Other types of arthrogryposis (congenital muscular dystrophy, neurogenic)
- Diagnosis
  - Prenatal ultrasound and MRI
- Prognosis
  - Most die in utero, at birth, or in neonatal period

References

Original:
Pena SD, Shokeir MH. Syndrome of camptodactyly, multiple ankyloses, facial anomalies, and pulmonary hypoplasia: a lethal condition. J Pediatr 1974;85:373–375.
Pena SD, Shokeir MH. Syndrome of camptodactyly, multiple ankyloses, facial anomalies and pulmonary hypoplasia-further delineation and evidence for autosomal recessive inheritance. Birth Defects Orig Artic Ser 1976;12:201–208.

Reviews and Case Reports:
Hall JG. Pena-Shokeir phenotype (fetal akinesia deformation sequence) revisited. Birth Defects Res A Clin Mol Teratol 2009 Aug;85(8):677–694.
Kalampokas E, Kalampokas T, Sofoudis C, Deligeeoroglou E, Botsis D. Diagnosing arthrogryposis multiplex congenita: a review. ISRN Obstet Gynecol 2012 Sep 23; Epub

Pendred Syndrome/DFNB4

(alt: Autosomal recessive sensorineural hearing impairment, Enlarged vestibular aqueduct and goiter)

- Organs Involved
  - Cochlear, vestibular aqueduct, thyroid gland

- Diagnostic Characteristics
  - Congenital sensorineural bilateral hearing loss (7.5 % of all cases of congenital deafness)
  - Hypothyroidism with goiter developing by age 10–20 years

- Associated Abnormalities
  - MRI of inner ear shows large vestibular aqueducts
  - Mondini dysplasia of cochleae
  - Hearing loss worsens over time and in relation to minor head trauma
  - Vertigo may occur after minor head trauma

- Genetics
  - Autosomal recessive inheritance
  - Mutations in the PDS gene, which codes for the pendrin protein, located on the long arm of chromosome 7 (7q31–34)

- Management
  - Avoid minor head trauma (e.g., contact sports)
  - Cochlear implants and speech and language support
  - Monitor thyroid hormone levels

References

Original:
Pendred V. Deaf-mutism and goiter. Lancet 1896;2:532.

Reviews and Case Reports:
Pearce JM. Pendred's syndrome. Eur Neurol 2007;58(3):189–190.
Reardon W, Coffey R, Phelps PD, et al. Pendred syndrome – 100 years of underascertainment. QJM 1997 July;90(7):443–447.
Bizhanova A, Kopp P. Genetics and phenomics of Pendred syndrome. Mol Cell Endocrinol 2010 Jun 30;322(1–2):83–90.

Perry Syndrome
(alt: Parkinsonism with alveolar hypoventilation and mental depression)

- Organs Involved
  - Substantia nigra, caudate nucleus, globus pallidus, medulla, respiratory
- Diagnostic Characteristics
  - Parkinsonism, early onset (mean age 48 years), familial
  - Hypoventilation
  - Depression
  - Weight loss
- Associated Abnormalities
  - Neuronal loss in substantia nigra, locus coeruleus, lentiform nucleus, hypothalamus, periaqueductal gray matter, and medulla
  - Sleep difficulties requiring ventilation support
- Prognosis
  - Response to levodopa usually poor; large doses required
  - Death within 10 years of onset

Genetics

Original:
Perry TL, Bratty PJ, Hansen S, Kennedy J, Urquhart N, Dolman CL. Hereditary mental depression and parkinsonism with taurine deficiency. Arch Neurol 1975;32:108–113.

Reviews and Case Reports:
Wszolek Z, Wider C. Perry syndrome. Parkinsonism with alveolar hypoventilation and mental depression. In: Pagon RA, Bird TD, Dolan CR, et al. editors. GeneReviews [internet], Seattle (WA): University of Washington, Seattle. 1993-Sep 30, 2010.

Purdy A, Hahn A, Barnett HJ, et al. Familial parkinsonism with alveolar hypoventilation and mental depression. Ann Neurol 1979 Dec;6(6):523–531.

Bhatia KP, Daniel SE, Marsden CD. Familial parkinsonism with depression: a clinicopathological study. Ann Neurol 1993 Dec;34(6):842–847.

Farrer MJ, Hulihan MM, Kachergus JM, et al. DCTN1 mutations in Perry syndrome. Nat Genet 2009 Feb;41(2):163–165.

Pfeiffer Syndrome Type 2
(alt: Acrocephalosyndactyly IV, V, and VI)

- ■ Organs Involved
  - • Skull, face, ears, teeth, digits

- ■ Diagnostic Characteristics
  - • Coronal synostosis, turribrachycephaly, cloverleaf-shaped head
  - • Hypertelorism, proptosis, maxillary hypoplasia
  - • Hearing loss
  - • Broad thumbs and great toes, syndactyly

- ■ Additional Abnormalities
  - • Cognitive defects in more severe forms
  - • Chiari type 1

- ■ Genetics
  - • Autosomal dominant inheritance, variable expressivity
  - • Frequent new mutations of fibroblast growth factor receptors 1 and 2
  - • Three subtypes: Type 1, normal intelligence, normal life span
  - • Type 2 and 3, more severe forms, type 2 with cloverleaf head

References

Original:
Pfeiffer RA. Dominante erbliche akrocephalosyndaktylie. Zeitschrift fur Kinderheilkunde, Berlin. 1964;90:301–320.
M Noack. Ein beitrag zum krankheitsbild der akrozephalosyndaktylie (Apert). Archiv fur Kinderheilkunde, Stuttgart. 1959;160:168–171.

Review and Case Reports:
Ranger A, Al-Hayek A, Matic D. Chiari type 1 malformation in an infant with type 2 Pfeiffer syndrome: further evidence of acquired pathogenesis. J Craniofac Surg 2010 Mar;21(2):427–431.

PHACES Syndrome
(alt: Posterior fossa malformation-hemangioma syndrome)

- Organs Involved
  - Brain-posterior fossa, skin of face, arteries, heart, eye (multiple congenital abnormalities)
- Diagnostic Characteristics
  - *P*osterior fossa and other brain abnormalities
  - *H*emangiomas of cervical facial region
  - *A*rterial cerebrovascular anomalies (congenital and/or progressive) (77 %)
  - *C*ardiac defects, aortic coarctation
  - *E*ye anomalies
  - *S*ternal defects
- Associated Abnormalities
  - Stroke in growth phase of infantile hemangioma 6–18 months
  - Seizures
  - Cortical dysgenesis
  - Headaches
  - Developmental delay
- Prognosis
  - Sometimes fatal, others improve after infancy

References

Original:
Frieden IJ, Reese V, Cohen D. PHACE syndrome. The association of posterior fossa brain malformations, hemangiomas, arterial anomalies, coarctation of the aorta and cardiac defects, and eye abnormalities. Arch Dermatol 1996 Mar;132(3):307–311.

Review and Case Reports:
Oza VS, Wang E, Berenstein A, et al. PHACES association: a neuroradiologic review of 17 patients. AJNR Am J Neuroradiol 2008 Apr;29(4):807–813.
Heyer GL, Dowling MM, Licht DJ, et al. The cerebral vasculopathy of PHACES syndrome. Stroke 2008 Feb;39(2):308–316.
Metry D, Heyer G, Hess C, et al. Consensus statement on diagnostic criteria for PHACE syndrome. Pediatrics 2009 Oct;124(5):1447–1456.

Phelan-Mcdermid Syndrome
(alt: 22q13.3 Deletion syndrome; Chromosome 22q13.3 deletion syndrome)

- Organs Involved
  - Muscles, face, head, brain

- Diagnostic Characteristics
  - Neonatal hypotonia
  - Delayed speech
  - Increased tolerance to pain
  - Global developmental delay
  - Moderate to severe intellectual impairment
  - Dolichocephaly
  - Ptosis, long eyelashes
  - Puffy cheeks, pointed chin
  - Large ears, large hands, thin toenails
  - Autistic-like affect, mouthing behavior, aversion to clothes
  - Chewing on clothing, toys, etc., hair pulling

- Genetics
  - Deletion of chromosome 22q13.3 involving gene SHANK3

- Differential Diagnosis
  - Angelman syndrome
  - Velocardiofacial syndrome
  - Fragile X syndrome

References

Original:
Phelan MC, Rogers RC, Saul RA, et al. 22q13 deletion syndrome. Am J Med Genet 2001;101(2):91–99.
Wilson HL, Wong AC, Shaw SR, et al. Molecular characterization of the 22q13 deletion syndrome supports the role of haploinsufficiency of SHANK3/PROSAP2 in the major neurological symptoms. J Med Genet 2003;40(8):575–584.

Reviews and Case Reports:
Phelan K, McDermid HE. The 22q13.3 deletion syndrome (Phelan-McDermid syndrome). Mol Syndromol 2012 Apr;2(3–5):186–201.
Phelan K, Rogers C. Phelan-McDermid syndrome. In: Pagon RA, Bird TD, Dolan CR, Stephens K, Adam MP. Editors, GeneReviews [internet]. Seattle (WA): University of Washington, Seattle; 1993–2005 May 11 [updated 2011 Aug 25]

Pitt-Hopkins Syndrome

- Organs Involved
  - Eyes, face, ears, brain, skull
- Diagnostic Characteristics
  - Facial features: deep-set eyes, strabismus, broad nasal bridge, large mouth, widely spaced teeth, ears with thick helix
  - Smiling disposition
  - Severe intellectual disability
  - Stereotypic movements of arms and fingers
  - Hypotonia, unsteady gait
  - Cryptorchidism
  - Intermittent hyperventilation followed by apnea and cyanosis
  - Microcephaly and seizures
- Associated Abnormalities
  - Hypoplastic corpus callosum, bulbous caudate nuclei
  - Slowing in EEG
  - Low levels of IgM
- Differential Diagnosis
  - Angelman syndrome
  - Mowat-Wilson syndrome
  - Rett syndrome
- Genetics
  - De novo mutations and insufficient expression of the TGF4 gene on long arm of chromosome 18 (18q21.2)

References

Original:
Pitt D, Hopkins I. A syndrome of mental retardation, wide mouth and intermittent overbreathing. Aust Paed J 1978;14(3):182–184.

Reviews and Case Reports:
Van Balkom ID, Vuijk PJ, Franssens M, Hoek HVV, Hennekam RC. Development, cognition, and behaviour in Pitt-Hopkins syndrome. Dev Med Chil Neurol 2012 Oct;54(10):925–931.
Zweier C, Peippo MM, Hoyer J, et al. Haploinsufficiency of TCF4 causes syndromal mental retardation with intermittent hyperventilation. (Pitt-Hopkins syndrome). Am J Hum Genet 2007 May;80(5):994–1001.

POEMS Syndrome

- Organs Involved
  - Peripheral nerves, endocrine glands, skin
- Diagnostic Characteristics
  - *P*olyneuropathy
  - *O*rganomegaly (liver, spleen, lymph nodes)
  - *E*ndocrinopathy or *e*dema
  - *M*-protein (IgG or IgA paraprotein)
  - *S*kin hyperpigmentation and hypertrichosis
- Associated Abnormalities
  - Papilledema
  - Pulmonary hypertension
  - Amenorrhoea in women, gynecomastia and testicular atrophy in men
  - Type 2 diabetes, hypothyroidism, adrenal insufficiency
  - Myeloma plasma-cell proliferative disorder in >50 % cases
- Criteria for Diagnosis
  - Required: polyneuropathy and monoclonal plasma-cell disorder, plus:
  - One major criterion (e.g., sclerotic bone lesion, elevated vascular endothelial growth factor)
  - One minor criterion (e.g., organomegaly, endocrinopathy, edema)
- Treatment
  - Steroids, IV immunoglobulin, and plasma exchange are usually ineffective.
  - Hematopoietic stem cell transplantation, variable effect.

References

Original:
Crow RS. Peripheral neuritis in myelomatosis. Br Med J 1956;2(4996):802–804.

Review and Case Reports:
Isose S, Misawa S, Kanai K, et al. POEMS syndrome with Guillain-Barre syndrome-like-acute onset: a case report and review of neurological progression in 30 cases. J Neurol Neurosurg Psychiatry 2011 Jun;82(6):678–680.

Poland Syndrome

- Organs Involved
  - Pectoralis muscle, fingers
- Diagnostic Characteristics
  - Underdevelopment or absence of pectoralis muscle, mostly right side and in males
  - Syndactyly of ipsilateral hand
- Associated Abnormalities
  - Dextrocardia
  - Diaphragmatic hernia
  - Absent radius
  - Absent nipple
  - Encephalocele
  - Microcephaly

References

Original:
Poland A. Deficiency of the pectoral muscles. Guy's Hosp Reports 1841;VI:191–193.
Clarkson P. Poland's syndactyly. Guys Hosp Rep 1962;111:335–346.

Review and Case Reports:
La Marca S, Delay E, Toussoun G, Ho Quoc C, Sinna R. Treatment of Poland syndrome thorax deformity with the lipomodeling technique: About 10 cases. Ann Chir Plast Esthet 2012 Nov 12; [Epub ahead of print]

Prader-Willi Syndrome

- Organs Involved
  - Muscles, face, skeleton, gonads, brain
- Diagnostic Characteristics
  - In utero: reduced fetal movements, polyhydramnios
  - Birth: breech or cesarean, hypotonia
  - Infancy: failure to thrive, delayed milestones, strabismus, cryptorchidism
  - Childhood: speech delay, hyperphagia, excessive weight gain
  - Adolescence: delayed puberty, short stature, obesity, scoliosis
  - Adulthood: hypogonadism, infertility, obesity, small hands and feet, borderline IQ, diabetes, learning and attention disorders, anxiety and OCD
- Genetics
  - Deletion of paternal copies of imprinted genes on chromosome 15 at 15q11–13 (Deletion of the same region on the maternal chromosome causes Angelman syndrome.)
- Differential Diagnosis
  - Down syndrome

References

Original:
Prader A, Labhart A, Willi H. Ein syndrome von adipositas, kleinwuchs, kryptorchismus und oligophrenie nach myatonleartigem zustand im neugeborenenalter. Schweizerische medizinische wochenschrift, Basel. 1956;86:1260–1261.

Review and Case Reports:
Holm VA, Cassidy SB, Butler MG, et al. Prader-Willi syndrome: consensus diagnostic criteria. Pediatrics 1993;91(2):398–402.
Benson LA, Maski KP, Kothare SV, Bourgeois BF. New onset epilepsy in Prader-Willi syndrome; semiology and literature review. Pediatr Neurol 2010 Oct;43(4):297–299.

Proteus Syndrome
(alt: Wiedemann syndrome)

- Organs Involved
  - Skin, bone, skull, brain
- Diagnostic Characteristics
  - Born normal, develop skin tumors and bone growths with increasing age
  - Skull, one or more limbs, and soles of feet especially affected by tissue overgrowth
  - Neurological involvement in rare reports of PS with hemimegalencephaly, Ohtahara syndrome, syringomyelia, arachnoid cyst, craniocutaneous lipomatosis, vascular malformation, and meningioma
- Genetics
  - Mutation in AKT1 kinase in a mosaic state gene
  - Classed as a genetic mosaicism

References

Original:
Temtamy S, Rogers J. Macrodactyly, hemihypertrophy, and connective tissue nevi; Report of a new syndrome and review of the literature. J Pediatr 1976 Dec;89(6):924–927.

Review and Case Reports:
Opitz J, Jorde. Hamartoma syndromes, exome sequencing, and a protean puzzle. N Engl J Med 2011 July 27;365(7):661–663.
Anik Y, Anik I, Gonullu E, Inan N, Demirci A. Proteus syndrome with syringohydromyelia and arachnoid cyst. Childs Nerv Syst 2007 Oct;23(10):1199–1202.
Bastos H, da Silva PF, de Albuquerque MA, et al. Proteus syndrome associated with hemimegalencephaly and Ohtahara syndrome: report of two cases. Seizure 2008 Jun;17(4):378–382.

R

Raeder's Paratrigeminal Syndrome – Russell-Silver Syndrome

Raeder's Paratrigeminal Syndrome
Ramsay Hunt Syndrome Type I
Ramsay Hunt Syndrome Type II
Rasmussen Syndrome
Renpenning Syndrome
Rett Syndrome
Reye Syndrome
Riley-Day Syndrome
Rosenberg-Chutorian Syndrome
Roussy-Levy Syndrome
Rubinstein-Taybi Syndrome
Russell-Silver Syndrome

J.G. Millichap, *Neurological Syndromes: A Clinical Guide to Symptoms and Diagnosis*, DOI 10.1007/978-1-4614-7786-0_17,
© Springer Science+Business Media New York 2013

Raeder's Paratrigeminal Syndrome
(alt: Raeder's paratrigeminal oculosympathetic syndrome)

- Organs Involved
  - Trigeminal nerve, oculosympathetic
- Diagnostic Characteristics
  - Severe unilateral facial pain and headache in the distribution of the ophthalmic division of the Vth trigeminal nerve
  - Unilateral oculosympathetic palsy (partial Horner syndrome)
  - Preservation of facial sweating
  - Lesion in middle cranial fossa, medial to trigeminal ganglion
- Causes
  - Carotid artery dissection
  - Carotid body tumor
  - Parasellar mass
  - Migraine headache
  - Vasculitis, sinusitis, osteitis
  - Head trauma
  - Hypertension

References

Original:
Raeder JG. Paratrigeminal paralysis of oculopupillary sympathetic. Brain 1924;47:149–158..

Review and Case Reports:
Klingon GH, Smith WM. Raeder's paratrigeminal syndrome. Neurology 1956;6(10):750–753.
Rao VA, Srinivasan R. Raeder's paratrigeminal syndrome. Indian J Ophthalmol 1981;29:59–61.
Murnane M, Proano L. Raeder's paratrigeminal syndrome: a case report. Acad Emerg Med 1996 Sep;3(9):864–867.

Ramsay Hunt Syndrome Type I
(alt: Dyssynergia cerebellaris myoclonica syndrome)

- Organs Involved
  - Cerebellum, cerebrum

- Diagnostic Characteristics
  - Action myoclonus presenting in first to second decade
  - Generalized epileptic seizures
  - Progressive cerebellar ataxia and tremor

- Associated Abnormalities
  - EEG fast generalized spike-and-wave discharges, photosensitivity, rolandic spikes during REM sleep

- Differential Diagnosis
  - Mitochondrial encephalomyopathy
  - Celiac disease
  - Neuronal ceroid lipofuscinosis (Batten disease)
  - Lafora body disease
  - Unverricht-Lundborg disease (stimulus-sensitive Baltic myoclonus)
  - Myoclonic epilepsy with ragged red fibers (muscle biopsy)
  - Spinocerebellar degenerative diseases

References

Original:
Hunt JR. Dyssynergia cerebellaris progressive: a chronic progressive form of cerebellar tremor. Brain 1914b;37(2):247.

Review and Case Reports:
Tassinari CA, Michelucci R, Genton P, Pellissier JF, Roger J. Dyssynergia cerebellaris myoclonica (Ramsay Hunt syndrome): a condition unrelated to mitochondrial encephalomyopathies. J Neurol Neurosurg Psychiatry 1989 Feb;52(2):262–265.
Lu CS, Thompson PD, Quinn NP, Parkes JD, Marsden CD. Ramsay Hunt syndrome and coeliac disease: a new association? Mov Disord 1986;1(3):209–219.

Ramsay Hunt Syndrome Type II
(alt: Herpes zoster oticus syndrome)

- Organs Involved
  - Geniculate ganglion, face, ear, tongue, vestibulocochlear nerve
- Diagnostic Characteristics
  - Acute facial nerve paralysis
  - Pain in the ear
  - Loss of taste, anterior 2/3rds of tongue
  - Dry mouth and eyes
  - Erythematous vesicular rash in the ear canal, tongue, and hard palate
- Associated Abnormalities
  - Tinnitus, hearing loss, vertigo
- Pathophysiology
  - Shingles of the geniculate ganglion
  - Illness that suppresses the immune system
- Prevention
  - Vaccination with Zostavax chickenpox vaccine
- Prognosis
  - Complete facial recovery in 75 % if treatment with prednisone and acyclovir started within first 3 days of onset. No recovery of hearing
  - Persistent facial paralysis in 50 % when treatment delayed

References

Original:
Hunt JR. On herpetic inflammations of the geniculate ganglion: a new syndrome and its complications. J Nerv Ment Dis 1907;34(2):73–96.

Review and Case Reports:
Murakami S, Hato N, Horiuchi J, Honda N, Gyo K, Yanagihara N. Treatment of Ramsay Hunt syndrome with acyclovir-prednisone: significance of early diagnosis and treatment. Ann Neurol 1997;41(3):353–357.

Rasmussen Syndrome
(alt: Rasmussen encephalitis; chronic focal encephalitis)

- Organs Involved
  - Cerebral hemisphere

- Diagnostic Characteristics
  - *Prodromal stage* of a few months. Children under 15 years of age
  - *Acute stage*, lasting 4–8 months, active inflammation
  - Hemiparesis, hemianopia, cognitive deficits
  - Focal motor seizures, partial or epilepsia partialis continua
  - *Chronic or residual stage,* seizures, hemiparesis, learning problems

- Diagnostic Tests
  - EEG slowing and seizure discharges over the affected hemisphere
  - MRI hemispheric cerebral atrophy with inflammation or scarring
  - Brain biopsy sometimes required

- Treatment
  - Steroids, antiepileptic medication
  - IV immunoglobulin
  - Plasmapheresis
  - Hemispherectomy in selected cases

References

Original:
Rasmussen T, Olszewski J, Lloyd-Smith D. Focal seizures due to chronic localized encephalitis. Neurology 1958;8(6):435–445.

Reviews and Case Reports:
Bien CG, Granata A. Pathogenesis, diagnosis and treatment of Rasmussen encephalitis: a European consensus statement. Brain 2005;128(Pt 3):454–471.
Hart YM, Cortez M, Andermann F, Hwang P, et al. Medical treatment of Rasmussen's syndrome (chronic encephalitis and epilepsy): effect of high-dose steroids or immunoglobulins in 19 patients. Neurology 1994 Jun;44(6):1030–1036.
Millichap JJ, Goldstein JL. Teaching neuroimages: long-term outcome of untreated Rasmussen syndrome. Neurology 2010 Nov 16;75(20):e85.

Renpenning Syndrome
(alt: Golabi-Ito-Hall syndrome; Sutherland-Haan syndrome)

- Organs Involved
  - Head, face, muscles, testes
- Diagnostic Characteristics
  - Regression in development at 3–4 years of age
  - Psychomotor retardation, hypotonia, and muscle atrophy
  - Microcephaly
  - Short stature
  - Facies long and narrow, bulbous nose, cup-shaped ears
  - Small testes
  - Seizures
- Associated Abnormalities
  - Coloboma
  - Cleft palate
  - Heart defect
- Genetics
  - Caused by mutations in the PQBP1 gene located on the X chromosome
  - X-linked recessive inheritance

References

Original:
Renpenning H, Gerrard JW, Zaleski WA, Tabata T. Familial sex-linked mental retardation. Can Med Assoc J 1962 Nov;87:954–956.

Review and Case Reports:
Stevenson RE, Bennett CW, Abidi F, et al. Renpenning syndrome comes into focus. Am J Med Genet A 2005 May 1;134(4):415–421.

Rett Syndrome

- ■ Organs Involved
  - • Brain gray matter

- ■ Diagnostic Characteristics
  - • Affects females almost exclusively; lethal in males
  - • Early deceleration of head growth
  - • Psychomotor regression phase aged 1–4 years followed by stabilization phase and late motor deterioration (50 % non-ambulant, nonverbal)
  - • Repetitive stereotyped hand movements (wringing, hands in mouth)
  - • Small hands and feet
  - • Seizures in ~80 %
  - • Rett syndrome is no longer listed in the new DSM-V, and is not classified as a form of autism. Rett syndrome is a genetic diagnosis, confirmed clinically and by MECP2 screening

- ■ Associated Abnormalities
  - • Scoliosis
  - • Growth failure
  - • Gastrointestinal disorders
  - • EEG abnormal in 80 %, mid-central spikes or sharp waves, enhanced by light sleep, pattern distinct from Angelman EEG

- ■ Genetics
  - • Mutations in gene MECP2 located on the X chromosome.
  - • Cause is a de novo mutation in 95 % cases and not inherited from either parent. X-linked dominant.
  - • Locus coeruleus, the source of noradrenergic innervation, is impaired by loss of MECP2, leading to low norepinephrine levels and symptoms of Rett syndrome.

References

Original:
Rett A. On an unusual brain atrophy syndrome in hyperammonemia in childhood. Wien Med Wochenschr 1966 Sep 10;116(37):723–726.

Review and Case Reports:
Percy AK. Rett syndrome: exploring the autism link. Arch Neurol 2011 Aug;68(8):985–989.
Jedele KB. The overlapping spectrum of Rett and Angelman syndromes: a clinical review. Semin Pediatr Neurol 2007 Sep;14(3):108–117.
Robb SA, Harden A, Boyd SG. Rett syndrome: an EEG study in 52 girls. Neuropediatrics 1989 Nov;20(4):192–195.

Reye Syndrome

- ■ Organs Involved
  - • Brain and liver
- ■ Diagnostic Characteristics – Five Stages
  - • Stage I. Rash, vomiting, confusion, fever, headaches
  - • Stage II. Encephalitis, hyperventilation, fatty liver, hyperreflexia
  - • Stage III. Coma, cerebral edema, respiratory arrest
  - • Stage IV. Deepening coma, fixed dilated pupils, hepatic dysfunction
  - • Stage V. Deep coma, seizures, multiple organ failure, hyperammonemia, severe brain and liver injury or death
- ■ Associated Abnormalities
  - • Aspirin ingestion
  - • Hypoglycemia
  - • Viral infection
- ■ Differential Diagnosis
  - • Inborn metabolic disorders
  - • Viral encephalitis
  - • Drug poisoning
  - • Head trauma
  - • Hepatic failure due to other causes
  - • Meningitis
  - • Renal failure
- ■ Preventive Precautions
  - • FDA recommends avoidance of aspirin containing products in children under 19 years of age during episodes of febrile illness, especially viral.

References

Original:
Reye RD, Morgan G, Baral J. Encephalopathy and fatty degeneration of the viscera. A disease entity in childhood. Lancet 1963;2(7311):749–752.

Review and Case Reports:
Starko KM, Ray CG, Dominguez LB, Stromberg WL, Woodall DF. Reye's syndrome and salicylate use. Pediatrics 1980 Dec;66(6):859–864.
Johnsen SD, Bird CR. The thalamus and midbrain in Reye syndrome. Pediatr Neurol 2006 May;34(5):405–407.
Singh P, Goraya JS, Gupta K, Saggar K, Ahluwalia A. Magnetic resonance imaging findings in Reye syndrome: case report and review of the literature. J Child Neurol 2011 Aug;26(8): 1009–1014.

Riley-Day Syndrome
(alt: Familial dysautonomia)

- Organs Involved
  - Autonomic nervous system, sensory neurons, eyes, tongue

- Diagnostic Characteristics
  - Congenital hypotonia and poor suck
  - Delayed milestones
  - Corneal irritation and absent tears
  - Blotchy skin
  - Unstable blood pressure
  - Insensitivity to pain, heat, and taste
  - Vomiting crises, dysphagia
  - Scoliosis

- Associated Abnormalities
  - Ashkenazi Jewish parents
  - Areflexia
  - Absent axon flare with intradermal histamine
  - Absent fungiform papillae on tongue

- Genetics
  - Autosomal recessive inheritance
  - Mutations in IKBKAP gene on chromosome 9

- Prognosis
  - Death by age 30 in 50 % from pneumonia or cardiopulmonary arrest

References

Original:
Riley CM, Day RL, Greely D, Langford WS. Central autonomic dysfunction with defective lacrimation. Pediatrics 1949;3(4):468–477.

Review and Case Reports:
Axelrod FB. Familial dysautonomia. Muscle Nerve 2004 Mar;29(3):352–363.
Gardiner J, Barton D, Vanslambrouck JM, et al. Defects in tongue papillae and taste sensation indicate a problem with neurotrophic support in various neurological diseases. Neuroscientist 2008 Jun;14(3):240–250.

Rosenberg-Chutorian Syndrome
(alt: Charcot-Marie-Tooth neuropathy X-linked recessive 5 (CMTX5))

- Organs Involved
  - Inner ear, auditory nerve, optic nerve, peripheral nerves
- Diagnostic Characteristics
  - Sensorineural deafness
  - Optic nerve atrophy
  - Peripheral neuropathy
- Genetics
  - Mutation in the PRPS1 gene located on X chromosome
  - Inherited as an X-linked disorder; males chiefly affected
- Differential Diagnosis
  - Iwashita syndrome (deafness, optic atrophy, polyneuropathy) – autosomal recessive inheritance
  - Hagemoser syndrome – autosomal dominant inheritance
  - Charcot-Marie-Tooth disease – autosomal dominant, recessive, or X-linked

References

Original:
Rosenberg RN, Chutorian A. Familial opticacoustic nerve degeneration and polyneuropathy. Neurology 1967;17:827–832.

Reviews and Case Reports:
Sugano M, Hirayama K, Saito T, Tsukamoto T, Yamamoto T. Optic atrophy, sensorineural hearing loss and polyneuropathy – a case of sporadic Rosenberg-Chutorian syndrome. Fukushima J Med Sci 1992 Jun;38(1):57–65.
Kim HJ, Sohn KM, Shy ME, et al. Mutations in PRPS1, which encodes the phosphoribosyl pyrophosphate synthetase enzyme critical for nucleotide biosynthesis, cause hereditary peripheral neuropathy with hearing loss and optic neuropathy (cmtx5). Am J Hum Genet 2007 Sep;81(3): 552–558.

Roussy-Levy Syndrome
(alt: Roussy-Levy hereditary areflexic dystasia)

- Organs Involved
  - Peripheral nerves, limb muscles, feet, spine

- Diagnostic Characteristics
  - Sensory gait ataxia
  - Pes cavus
  - Areflexia
  - Loss of vibration and position sense
  - Muscle atrophy in the legs
  - Postural tremor
  - Kyphoscoliosis

- Course and Prognosis
  - Onset in infancy and course relatively benign
  - Chronic demyelinating neuropathy with hypertrophic myelin sheath

- Genetics
  - Similar to the demyelinating type of Charcot-Marie-Tooth disease, CMT-1B with onion-bulb formation
  - Mutations in the myelin protein genes P0, 22, and MPZ
  - No cerebellar degeneration but clinically similar to Friedreich's ataxia and only distinguished by genetic testing

References

Original:
Plante-Bordeneuve V, Guiochon-Mantel A, Lacroix C, Lapresle J, Said G. The Roussy-Levy family: from the original description to the gene. Ann Neurol 1999 Nov;46(5):770–773.
Patzko A, Shy ME. Charcot-Marie-Tooth disease and related genetic neuropathies. Continuum (Minneap Minn) 2012 Feb;18(1):39–59.

Rubinstein-Taybi Syndrome
(alt: Broad thumb-hallux syndrome)

- Organs Involved
  - Thumbs, toes, face, head, testes
- Diagnostic Characteristics
  - Broad thumbs and broad first toes
  - Learning disability, mental retardation
  - Dysmorphic features, prominent beaked nose
  - Microcephaly, microphthalmia
  - Short stature
- Associated Abnormalities
  - Adverse reactions to anesthesia or succinylcholine
- Genetics
  - Mutations in the CREBBP gene (and EP300 gene)

References

Original:
Rubinstein JH, Taybi H. Broad thumbs and toes and facial abnormalities. A possible mental retardation syndrome. Am J Dis Child 1963 Jun;105:588–608.

Review and Case Reports:
Kumar S, Suthar R, Panigrahi I, Manwaha RK. Rubinstein-Taybi syndrome: Clinical profile of 11 patients and review of literature. Indian J Hum Genet 2012 May;18(2):161–166.

Russell-Silver Syndrome

- ■ Organs Involved
  - • Head, face, body, limbs

- ■ Diagnostic Characteristics
  - • Intrauterine growth restriction, dwarfism
  - • Low birth weight
  - • Feeding problems
  - • Triangular face
  - • Large head, relative macrocephaly
  - • Body asymmetry, hemihypertrophy
  - • Hypotonia

- ■ Etiology
  - • Maternal uniparental disomy on chromosome 7 in 5–10 %
  - • Hypomethylation on chromosome 11p15 in ~60 %
  - • Genomic imprinting disorder

References

Original:
Russell A. A syndrome of intra-uterine dwarfism recognizable at birth with cranio-facial dysostosis, disproportionately short arms, and other anomalies (5 examples). Proc R Soc Med 1954;47(12):1040–1044.
Silver HK, Kiyasu W, George J, Deamer WC. Syndrome of congenital hemihypertrophy, shortness of stature, and elevated urinary gonadotropins. Pediatrics 1953;12(4):368–376.

Review and Case Reports:
Eggermann T. Russell-Silver syndrome. Am J Med Genet C Semin Med Genet 2010 Aug 15;154C(3):355–364.
Wakeling EL. Silver-Russell syndrome. Arch Dis Child 2011 Dec;96(12):1156–1161.

S

Saethre-Chotzen Syndrome – Susac Syndrome

Saethre-Chotzen Syndrome
Sandifer Syndrome
Satoyoshi Syndrome
Schimmelpenning-Feuerstein-Mims Syndrome
Schneider Syndrome
Schwartz-Bartter Syndrome
Schwartz-Jampel Syndrome Type IA
Septo-Optic Dysplasia
Serotonin Syndrome
Shapiro Syndrome
Shprintzen-Goldberg Syndrome
Shy-Drager Syndrome
Simpson-Golabi-Behmel Syndrome Type 1
Sjogren-Larsson Syndrome
Smith-Lemli-Opitz Syndrome
Smith-Magenis Syndrome
Sotos Syndrome
Stickler Syndrome
Stiff Person Syndrome
Strachan Syndrome
Sturge-Weber Syndrome
SUCLA2 Deficiency Syndrome
Susac Syndrome

J.G. Millichap, *Neurological Syndromes: A Clinical Guide to Symptoms and Diagnosis*, DOI 10.1007/978-1-4614-7786-0_18, © Springer Science+Business Media New York 2013

Saethre-Chotzen Syndrome
(alt: Acrocephalosyndactyly type III syndrome)

- ■ Organs Involved
  - • Skull, face, eyes, ears, fingers
- ■ Diagnostic Characteristics
  - • Coronal synostosis, brachycephaly, acrocephaly
  - • Facial asymmetry
  - • Ptosis, strabismus, and small ear pinna
  - • Syndactyly
- ■ Associated Abnormalities
  - • Vertebral fusions
  - • Ocular hypertelorism
  - • Congenital heart malformations
- ■ Genetics
  - • Mutations in the TWIST1 gene on chromosome 7 involving 7p21
  - • Autosomal dominant inheritance
- ■ Differential Diagnosis of Autosomal Craniosynostosis Syndromes
  - • Apert syndrome
  - • Vogt syndrome
  - • Waardenburg syndrome
  - • Pfeiffer syndrome
  - • Muenke syndrome

References

Original:
Saethre H. Ein beitrag zum turmschadelproblem (pathogenese, erblichkeit und symptomologie). Dtsch z Nervenheilkd 1931;117:533–555.
Chotzen F. Eine eigenartige familiare entwicklungsstorung. (Akrocephalosyndaktylie, dystosis craniofacialis und hypertelorismus). Monatschr Kinderheilkd 1932;55:97–122.

Review and Case Reports:
Spaggiari E, Aboura A, Sinico M, et al. Prenatal diagnosis of a 7p15-p21 deletion encompassing the TWIST1 gene involved in Saethre-Chotzen syndrome. Eur J Med Genet 2012 Aug-Sep;55(8–9):498–501.
Zechi-Ceide RM, Rodrigues MG, Jehee FS, Kokitsu-Nakata NM, Passos-Bueno MR, Guion-Almeida ML. Saethre-Chotzen phenotype with learning disability and hyper IgE phenotype in a patient due to complex chromosomal rearrangement involving chromosomes 3 and 7. Am J Med Genet A 2012 Jul;158A(7):1680–1685.
Gallagher ER, Ratisoontorn CV, Cunningham ML. Saethre-Chotzen syndrome. In: Pagon RA, Bird TD, Dolan CR, et al. editors. GeneReviews [internet]. Seattle (WA): University of Washington, Seattle; 1993- June 14, 2012.
Clauser L, Galle M. Saethre-Chotzen syndrome. Orphanet Encyclopedia, Edited by Hennekam RCM. July 2004.

Sandifer Syndrome

- Organs Involved
  - Gastroesophageal junction, neck, limbs
- Diagnostic Characteristics
  - Gastroesophageal reflux (GERD)
  - Spastic torticollis
  - Dystonic body movements
  - Hiatal hernia
- Treatment
  - Medical for GERD
  - Surgical fundoplication for hiatal hernia

References

Original:
Kinsbourne M. Hiatus hernia with contortions of the neck. Lancet 1964;1:1058–1061.

Review and Case Reports:
Lehwald N, Krausch M, Franke C, Assmann B, Adam R, Knoefel WT. Sandifer syndrome – a multidisciplinary diagnostic and therapeutic challenge. Eur J Pediatr Surg 2007 Jun;17(3):203–206.
Nowak M, Strzelczyk A, Oertel WH, Hamer HM, Rosenow F. A female adult with Sandifer's syndrome and hiatal hernia misdiagnosed as epilepsy with focal seizures. Epilepsy Behav 2012 May;24(1):141–142.

Satoyoshi Syndrome
(alt: Komura-Guerri syndrome)

- ■ Organs Involved
  - • Muscle, hair, intestine, uterus, skeleton
- ■ Diagnostic Characteristics
  - • Progressive painful muscle spasms beginning in lower limbs and thumbs, onset 6–15 years of age, and later involving the pectoral girdle, trunk, and finally the masseters and temporal muscles
  - • Alopecia
  - • Diarrhea
  - • Endocrinopathy: amenorrhea and uterine hypoplasia
  - • Growth failure after 10–12 years of age
- ■ Etiology and Treatment
  - • Autoimmune disorder likely
  - • Prednisolone, methotrexate, and carbamazepine found of benefit

References

Original:
Satoyoshi E, Yamada K. Recurrent muscle spasms of central origin. A report of two cases. Neurology 1967;28:456–471.

Review and Case Reports:
Heger S, Kuester RM, Volk R, Stephani U, Sippell WG. Satoyoshi syndrome: a rare multisystemic disorder requiring systemic and symptomatic treatment. Brain Dev 2006 Jun;26(5):300–304.
Drost G, Verrips A, van Engelen BG, Stegeman DF, Zwarts MJ. Involuntary painful muscle contractions in Satoyoshi syndrome: a surface electromyographic study. Mov Disord 2006 Nov;21(11):2015–2018.

Schimmelpenning-Feuerstein-Mims Syndrome
(Linear nevus sebaceous syndrome; Solomon syndrome)

- ■ Organs Involved
  - • Brain, skin, eye, skeleton, heart, kidney
- ■ Diagnostic Characteristics
  - • Sebaceus nevus
  - • Mental retardation
  - • Seizures
  - • Hemimegalencephaly, gyral malformations
  - • Eye abnormalities: coloboma, choristomas
  - • Scoliosis
- ■ Genetics
  - • Mutations in HRAS and KRAS genes
  - • Probably autosomal dominant
  - • Frequently sporadic rather than inherited
- ■ Investigations Indicated
  - • MRI, skeletal survey, EEG

References

Original:
Schimmelpenning G. Klinischer beitrag zur symptomatology der phacomatosen. Fortschr Roentgenstr 1957;57(6):716.
Feuerstein RC, Mims LC. Linear nevus sebaceus with convulsions and mental retardation. Amer J Dis Child 1962;104:674–679.

Review and Case Reports:
Menascu S, Donner EJ. Linear nevus sebaceous syndrome: case reports and review of the literature. Pediatr Neurol 2008;38(3):207.
Hsieh CW, Wu YH, Lin SP, Peng CC, Ho CS. Sebaceous nevus syndrome, central nervous system malformations, aplasia cutis congenita, limbal dermoid, and pigmented nevus syndrome. Pediatr Dermatol 2012 May-Jun;29(3):365–367.

Schneider Syndrome
(alt: Central cord syndrome)

- Organs Involved
  - Cervical spinal cord

- Diagnostic Characteristics
  - Acute cervical spinal cord injury with incomplete paralysis
  - Greater motor loss in upper extremities compared to lower
  - Sensory impairment below level of injury
  - Bladder dysfunction and urinary retention

- Causes
  - Occurs with spinal hyperextension injury in older individual with cervical spondylosis
  - May occur with trauma and/or bleeding in central part of cord in younger individuals
  - Complication of generalized tonic clonic seizure or status epilepticus

- Prognosis
  - Generally favorable for some degree of recovery, dependent on age and extent of injury

References

Original:
Schneider RC, Cherry G, Pantek H. The syndrome of acute central cervical spinal cord injury; with special reference to the mechanisms involved in hyperextension injuries of cervical spine. J Neurosurg 1954;11(6):546–577.

Review and Case Reports:
Lee S, Lee JE, Yang S, Chang H. A case of central cord syndrome related status epilepticus – a case report-. Ann Rehabil Med 2011 Aug;35(4):574–578.
Yadla S, Klimo P, Harrop JS. Traumatic central cord syndrome: etiology, management, and outcomes. Topics in Spinal Cord Injury Rehabilitation 2010;15(3):73–84.

Schwartz-Bartter Syndrome
(alt: Inappropriate secretion of antidiuretic hormone syndrome)

- Organs Involved
  - Antidiuretic hormone

- Diagnostic Characteristics
  - Inappropriate secretion of antidiuretic hormone
  - Headache, confusion, disorientation, hostility, and progressive memory impairment without motor or sensory deficits
  - Absence of dehydration or edema and no signs of renal, hepatic, or cardiac disease

- Associated Abnormalities
  - Vasopressin secreting tumors
  - Small cell and oat-cell lung carcinomas
  - HHV-6 infection with acute limbic encephalitis

References

Original:
Schwartz WB, Bennett W, Curelop S, Bartter FC. A syndrome of renal sodium loss and hyponatremia probably resulting from inappropriate secretion of antidiuretic hormone. Am J Medicine, New York, 1957;23:529–542.

Review and Case Reports:
Kawaguchi T, Takeuchi M, Kawajiri C, et al. Severe hyponatremia caused by syndrome of inappropriate secretion of antidiuretic hormone developed as initial manifestation of human herpesvirus-6-associated acute limbic encephalitis after unrelated bone marrow transplantation. Transpl Infect Dis 2012 Nov 23.doi:10.1111/tid 12029. [Epub ahead of print].
Graziani G, Cucchiari D, Aroldi A, Angelini C, Gaetani P, Selmi C. Syndrome of inappropriate secretion of antidiuretic hormone in traumatic brain injury: when tolvaptan becomes a life saving drug. J Neurol Neurosurg Psychiatry 2012 May;83(5):510–512.
Blondin NA, Vortmeyer AO, Harel NY. Paraneoplastic syndrome of inappropriate antidiuretic hormone mimicking limbic encephalitis. Arch Neurol 2011 Dec;68(12):1591–1594.

Schwartz-Jampel Syndrome Type IA

- Organs Involved
  - Muscles, nerves, face, joints, spine, chest
- Diagnostic Characteristics
  - Muscle stiffness (myotonia) at birth
  - Short stature
  - Flattened facies, micrognathia, blepharophimosis, microstomia
  - Short neck, kyphosis, pectus carinatum
- Associated Abnormalities
  - Elevated creatine kinase and lactic dehydrogenase
  - EMG generalized myotonia
- Genetics
  - Autosomal recessive transmission
  - Causative gene HSPG2 on chromosome 1p34–p36
- Differential Diagnosis
  - Stuve-Wiedemann disease (no gene defect recognized)
  - Congenital myotonia
- Treatment
  - Myotonia may respond to carbamazepine
- Prognosis
  - Disease stabilizes after adolescence.

References

Original:
Schwartz O, Jampel RS. Congenital blepharophimosis associated with a unique generalized myopathy. Arch Ophthalmol !962 Jul;68:52–57.

Review and Case Reports:
Zhang S, Wu HS, Lu JL. Clinical analysis of four patients with Schwartz-Jampel syndrome. Zhonghua Er Ke Za Zhi 2012 Mar;50(3):231–234.
Regalo SC, Vitti M, Semprini M, et al. The effect of the Schwartz-Jampel syndrome on masticatory and facial musculatures-an electromyographic analysis. Electromyogr Clin Neurophysiol 2005 Apr-May;45(3):183–189.

Septo-Optic Dysplasia
(alt: de Morsier syndrome)

- Organs Involved
  - Optic nerves, pituitary gland, septum pellucidum

- Diagnostic Characteristics
  - Optic nerve hypoplasia
  - Absent septum pellucidum
  - Hypopituitarism, growth hormone deficiency

- Associated Abnormalities
  - Congenital nystagmus, small optic disc, hyperplastic vitreous
  - Variable visual impairment
  - Digital defects
  - Hyperbilirubinemia
  - Seizures
  - In utero drug exposure (cocaine, valproate, recreational)
  - Heterotopias, arachnoid cysts

- Genetics
  - Sporadic birth defect of unknown cause
  - HESX1 mutations are uncommon cause

- Treatment
  - Hormone replacement therapy

References

Original:
de Morsier G. Etudes sur les dysgraphies, cranioencephaliques III. Agenesie du septum palludicum avec malformation du tractus optique. La dysplasie septo-optique. Schweizer Archiv fur Neurologie und Psychiatrie, Zurich 1956;77:267–292.

Review and Case Report:
Webb EA, Dattani MT. Septo-optic dysplasia. Eur J Hum Genet 2010 Apr;18(4):393–397.
Tas E, Tracy M, Sarco DP, Eksioglu YZ, Prabhu SP, Loddenkemper T. Septo-optic dysplasia complicated by infantile spasms and bilateral choroidal fissure arachnoid cysts. J Neuroimaging 2011 Jan;21(1):89–91.

Serotonin Syndrome
(alt: Serotonin toxicity)

- Organs Involved
  - CNS serotonin receptors
- Signs and Symptoms (Clinical Triad)
  - *Cognitive effects*: headache, agitation, hypomania, confusion, hallucinations, coma
  - *Autonomic effects*: shivering, seating, hyperthermia, hypertension, tachycardia, nausea, diarrhea
  - *Somatic effects*: myoclonus, hyperreflexia, clonus, tremor
- Diagnostic Characteristics (Hunter Criteria)
  - Spontaneous clonus
  - Inducible clonus plus agitation or diaphoresis
  - Ocular clonus plus agitation or diaphoresis
  - Tremor plus hyperreflexia
  - Hypertonism plus temperature > 38 C (100 F) plus ocular clonus or inducible clonus
- Cause
  - Ingestion of serotonergic medications in high dose or combination: MAO inhibitor antidepressants, CNS stimulants, triptans, L-Dopa, lithium.
  - Overstimulation of the 5-HT receptors.
  - Noradrenergic CNS hyperactivity may play a role.
- Differential Diagnosis
  - Neuroleptic malignant syndrome (dopamine receptor blockade) (bradykinesia and rigidity in NMS, hyperkinesia and clonus in SS)

References

Original:
Oates JA, Sjoerdsma A. Neurologic effects of tryptophan in patients receiving a monoamine oxidase inhibitor. Neurology 1960 Dec;10:1076–1078.

Review and Case Reports:
Boyer EW, Shannon M. The serotonin syndrome. N Engl J Med 2005;352(11):1112–1120.
Dunkley EJ, Isbister GK, Sibbritt D, Dawson AH, Whyte IM. The Hunter Serotonin Toxicity Criteria: simple and accurate diagnostic decision rules for serotonin toxicity. QJM 2003 Sep;96(9):635–642.

Shapiro Syndrome
(alt: Spontaneous periodic hypothermia and hyperhidrosis)

- Organs Involved
  - Hypothalamus

- Diagnostic Characteristics
  - Paroxysmal hypothermia, with hyperhidrosis, adult onset, variable frequency, hours to weeks to years
  - Agenesis of the corpus callosum

- Treatment
  - Anticonvulsants, clonidine, cyproheptadine

- Causes Postulated
  - Unknown
  - Diencephalic epilepsy (but EEG normal)
  - Dysfunctional thermoregulatory center in hypothalamus

References

Original:
Shapiro WR, Williams GH, Plum F. Spontaneous recurrent hypothermia accompanying agenesis of the corpus callosum. Brain 1969;92:423–436.

Review and Case Reports:
Kloos RT. Spontaneous periodic hypothermia. Medicine (Baltimore) 1995 Sep;74(5):268–280.
Dundar NO, Boz A, Duman O, Aydin F, Haspolat S. Spontaneous periodic hypothermia and hyperhidrosis. Pediatr Neurol 2008 Dec;39(6):438–440.
Tambasco N, Corea F, Bocola V. Subtotal corpus callosum agenesis with recurrent hyperhidrosis-hypothermia (Shapiro syndrome). Neurology 2005 Jul 12;65(1):124.
Sheth RD, Barron TF, Hartlage PL. Episodic spontaneous hypothermia with hyperhidrosis: implications for pathogenesis. Pediatr Neurol 1994 Feb;10(1):58–60.

Shprintzen-Goldberg Syndrome
(alt: Marfanoid-Craniosynostosis syndrome)

- Organs Involved
  - Skull, face, fingers, spine, brain, heart
- Diagnostic Characteristics
  - Craniosynostosis
  - Dolichocephaly, prominent forehead
  - Ocular proptosis, hypertelorism, downslanting palpebral fissures
  - Maxillary hypoplasia, micrognathia, low-set ears
  - Arachnodactyly, pectus exavatum, scoliosis
  - Mitral valve prolapse
  - Delayed psychomotor development
  - Hydrocephalus, Chiari type 1 malformation
- Associated Abnormalities
  - C1–C2 abnormality, wide anterior fontanel, 13 pairs of ribs on X-ray
- Genetics
  - Mutations in FBN1 in some cases
  - Mode of inheritance unknown

References

Original:
Shprintzn RJ, Goldberg RB. A recurrent pattern syndrome of craniosynostosis associated with arachnodactyly and abdominal hernias. J Craniofac Genet Dev Biol 1982;2:65–74.

Review and Case Reports:
Greally MT, Crey JC, Milewicz DM, et al. Shprintzen-Goldberg syndrome: a clinical analysis. Am J Med Genet 1998 Mar 19;76(3):202–212.
Greally MT. Shprintzen-Goldberg syndrome. In: Pagon RA, Bird TD, Dolan CR, et al., editors. GeneReviews [internet], Seattle (WA): University of Washington, Seattle, 1993- Update Nov 16, 2010.

Shy-Drager Syndrome
(alt: Multiple system atrophy)

- ■ Organs Involved
  - ● Autonomic nervous system, cerebellum, striatonigral system
- ■ Diagnostic Characteristics
  - ● Autonomic dysfunction
  - ● Parkinsonism
  - ● Ataxia
- ■ Associated Abnormalities
  - ● Orthostatic hypotension
  - ● Urinary incontinence
  - ● Vocal cord paralysis
  - ● Sleep apnea
- ■ Pathology
  - ● Abundant glial and neuronal cytoplasmic inclusions (Papp-Lantos bodies) in CNS are defining histopathologic hallmark of multiple system atrophy.
- ■ Prognosis
  - ● Average life span of 8 years after symptom onset.
  - ● Most patients are disabled within 5 years of onset.
- ■ Treatment
  - ● Symptomatic, especially avoidance of triggers of hypotension.
  - ● Poor response to L-Dopa is a characteristic.

References

Original:
Shy GM, Drager GA. A neurological syndrome associated with orthostatic hypotension: a clinical-pathological study. Arch Neurol 1960;2:511–527.

Review and Case Reports:
Gillman S, Wenning GK, Low PA, et al. Second consensus statement on the diagnosis of multiple system atrophy. Neurology 2008;71(9):670–676.

Simpson-Golabi-Behmel Syndrome Type 1

- Organs Involved
  - Craniofacial, tongue, palate, umbilicus, heart, diaphragm, skeleton
- Diagnostic Characteristics
  - Macrosomia, macrocephaly
  - Hypertelorism, downslanting palpebral fissures
  - Dysmorphic facial features, broad nose ("bulldog" facies)
  - Macrostomia, macroglossia
  - Furrowed tongue and lower lip
  - Cleft lip and/or palate
  - Micrognathia in neonates, macrognathia in older individuals
  - Mild to severe intellectual disability
- Associated Abnormalities
  - Umbilical hernia, GI, and genitourinary anomalies
  - Congenital heart defects
  - Skeletal anomalies, scoliosis
  - Polydactyly and large hands
  - Increased risk of embryonal tumors (Wilms, adrenal, etc.)
- Genetics
  - X-linked inheritance; males are affected, female carriers.
  - Mutations in GPC3 and GPC4 genes on Xq26.

References

Original:

Simpson JL, Landey S, New M, German J. A previously unrecognized X-linked syndrome of dysmorphia. Birth Defects Orig Artic Ser 1975;11:18–24.

Golabi M, Rosen L. A new X-linked mental retardation-overgrowth syndrome. Am J Med Genet 1984;17:345–358.

Behmel A, Plochi E, Rosenkranz W. A new X-linked dysplasia gigantism syndrome: identical with the Simpson dysplasia syndrome? Hum Genet 1984;67:409–413.

Review and Case Reports:

Young EL, Wishnow R, Nigro MA. Expanding the clinical picture of Simpson-Golabi-Behmel syndrome. Pediatr Neurol 2006 Feb;34(2):139–142.

Sjogren-Larsson Syndrome

- ■ Organs Involved
  - • Skin, lower limbs, brain
- ■ Diagnostic Characteristics
  - • Congenital ichthyosis
  - • Spastic paraparesis
  - • Mental retardation
- ■ Genetics
  - • Autosomal recessive inherited disorder of lipid metabolism
  - • ALDH gene mutations on chromosome 17
  - • Associated with deficiency of the enzyme fatty aldehyde dehydrogenase

References

Original:
Sjogren T, Larsson T. Oligophrenia in combination with congenital ichthyosis and spastic disorders: a clinical and genetic study. Acta Psychiatr Neurol Scand Suppl 1957;113:1–112.

Review and Case Reports:
Davis K, Holden KR, S'aulis D, Amador C, Matheus MG, Rizo WB. Novel mutation in Sjogren-Larsson syndrome is associated with divergent neurologic phenotypes. J Child Neurol 2012 Oct 3;[Epub ahead of print]
Fuijkschot J, Theelen T, Seyger MM, et al. Sjogren-Larrsson syndrome in clinical practice. J Inherit Metab Dis 2012 Nov;35(6):955–962.

Smith-Lemli-Opitz Syndrome
(alt: SLO syndrome; 7-dehydrocholesterol reductase deficiency)

- Organs Involved
  - Face, head, fingers and toes, palate, brain
- Diagnostic Characteristics
  - Dysmorphic face
  - Prenatal and postnatal growth retardation
  - Microcephaly
  - Intellectual impairment
  - Cleft palate
  - Low blood level of 7-dehydrocholesterol
- Genetics
  - Autosomal recessive inheritance
  - Mutations in the DHCR7 gene with 7-DHC-reductase deficiency

References

Original:
Smith DW, Lemli L, Opitz JM. A newly recognized syndrome of multiple congenital anomalies. J Pediatr, St Louis 1964;64:210–217.

Review and Case Reports:
Opitz JM, de la Cruz F. Cholesterol metabolism in the RSH/Smith-Lemli-Opitz syndrome: Summary of an NICHD conference. Am J Med Genet, New York 1994;50:326–338.
Opitz JM. RSH/SLO (Smith-Lemli-Opitz) syndrome: Historical, genetic and developmental considerations. Am J Med Genet, New York 1994;50:344–346.
Irons M. Smith-Lemli-Opitz syndrome. In: Pagon RA, Bird TD, Dolan CR, et al., editors. GeneReviews [internet], Seattle (WA): University of Washington, Seattle; 1993- update Oct 24, 2007.

Smith-Magenis Syndrome

- Organs Involved
  - Face, muscle, skeleton, fingers, peripheral nerves, eyes

- Diagnostic Characteristics
  - Distinctive facial features: broad, square face with deep-set eyes
  - Prognathism, more marked in later childhood
  - Inverted sleep rhythms, sleepy during the day and awakens at night
  - Behavioral problems, sometimes pleasant, frequently impulsive, inattentive, and aggressive
  - Self-injury, biting, head banging, and skin picking very common
  - Self-hugging, "lick and flip" pages of books, unique behaviorisms
  - Recall trivia about people and subjects

- Associated Abnormalities
  - Short stature, scoliosis
  - Reduced sensitivity to pain and temperature
  - Myopia, strabismus
  - Rare heart and kidney defects

- Genetics
  - Deletion or mutation of RAI1 gene on chromosome 17 at 17p11.2

References

Original:
Smith ACM, McGavran L, Waldstein G. Deletion of the 17 short arm in two patients with facial clefts. Am J Hum Genet, Chicago 1982;34 (Suppl):A410.
Smith ACM, McGavran L, Robinson J, Waldstein G, Macfarlane J, Zonana J, Reiss J, Lahr M, Allen L, Magenis E. Interstitial deletion of 17 (p11.2) in nine patients. Am J Med Genet, New York 1986;24:393–414.

Review and Case Reports:
Gropman AL, Elsea S, Duncan WC Jr, Smith AC. New developments in Smith-Magenis syndrome (del 17p11.2). Curr Opin Neurol 2007 Apr;20(2):125–134.
Gropman AL, Duncan WC, Smith AC. Neurologic and developmental features of the Smith-Magenis syndrome (del 17p11.2). Pediatr Neurol 2006 May;34(5):337–350.

Sotos Syndrome
(alt: Cerebral gigantism)

- Organs Involved
  - Head, face, body, limbs, muscles

- Diagnostic Characteristics
  - Macrosomia at birth
  - Advanced bone age and growth rate in childhood
  - Macrocephaly
  - Macrodactyly
  - Hypertelorism
  - Mild intellectual impairment
  - Delayed psychomotor development, learning disabilities
  - Hypotonia
  - *Major diagnostic criteria*: facial gestalt, early growth excess, advanced bone age, early developmental delay, normalization of growth rate after first few years, and improved cognitive development in school age and adulthood

- Associated Abnormalities
  - Speech impairment
  - Awkward gait, incoordination
  - Behavior disorder, aggressiveness, irritability
  - Congenital heart defects
  - Scoliosis
  - Seizures

- Genetics
  - Mutations involving the NSD1 gene on chromosome 5
  - Familial cases rare. Most occur sporadically

References

Original:
Sotos JE, Dodge PR, Muirhead D, Crawford JD, Talbot NB. Cerebral gigantism in childhood. A syndrome of excessively rapid growth and acromegalic features and a nonprogressive neurologic disorder. N Engl J Med 1964 Jul 16;271:109–116.
Schlesinger B. Gigantism (acromegalic in type). Proc R Soc Med 1931;24:1352–1353.

Review and Case Reports:
Cole TR, Hughes HE. Sotos syndrome: a study of the diagnostic criteria and natural history. J Med Genet 1994 Jan;31(1):20–32.
Leventopoulos G, Kitsiou-Tzeli S, Kritikos K, et al. A clinical study of Sotos syndrome patients with review of the literature. Pediatr Neurol 2009 May;40(5):357–364.

Stickler Syndrome

- Organs Involved
  - Connective tissue, joints, face, palate, eyes, inner ear
- Diagnostic Characteristics
  - Flattened facial features
  - Pierre Robin sequence (cleft palate, micrognathia, and glassoptosis)
  - Myopia, glaucoma, retinal detachment, cataract
  - Arthritis, scoliosis, hypermobile joints
  - Sensorineural and conductive hearing impairment
  - Learning difficulties
- Genetics
  - Mutations in the COL11A genes involved in collagen formation
  - Autosomal dominant trait with variable expressivity and incomplete penetrance

References

Original:
Stickler GB, Belau PG, Farrel FJ, et al. Hereditary progressive arthro-ophthalmopathy. Mayo Clin Proc, Rochester, MN. 1965;40:433–455.

Review and Case Reports:
Nowack CB. Genetics and hearing loss: a review of Stickler syndrome. J Commun Disord 1998;31(5):437–453.

Stiff Person Syndrome
(alt: Stiff-man syndrome; Stiff baby syndrome; Moersch-Woltman Condition)

- Organs Involved
  - Axial muscles
- Diagnostic Characteristics
  - Stiffness and pain in the back
  - Muscle spasms in response to environmental stimuli
  - Exaggerated lumbar lordosis
  - Occurs in adults (30–50 years of age) and in young children
- Associated Abnormalities
  - Hypertonia, hyperreflexia, muscle rigidity
  - Increased startle and head retraction reflexes
- Causes
  - Autoimmune cause suggested by occurrence of circulating antibodies to the enzyme glutamic acid decarboxylase (GAD65)
  - Mutation in GLRA1 (glycine receptor) gene responsible in some cases
- Differential Diagnosis
  - Tetanus
  - Hyperekplexia
  - Strychnine poisoning
  - Neuromyotonia (Isaac syndrome)
- Treatment
  - Muscle relaxants which potentiate GABA (benzodiazepines)
  - IV immunoglobulin, azathioprine, prednisone, or cyclophosphamide
  - Plasmapheresis
  - Monoclonal antibody rituximab

References

Original:
Moersch FP, Woltman HW. Progressive fluctuating muscular rigidity and spasm ("stiff-man" syndrome); report of a case and some observations in 13 other cases. Mayo Clin Proc 1956;31(15): 421–427.

Review and Case Reports:
McKeon A, Robinson MT, McEvoy KM, et al. Stiff-man syndrome and variants: clinical course, treatments, and outcomes. Arch Neurol 2012 Feb;69(2):230–238.

Strachan Syndrome
(alt: Jamaican neuritis; Cuban neuropathy; nutritional neuropathy)

- ■ Organs Involved
  - Peripheral nerves, optic nerves

- ■ Diagnostic Characteristics
  - Pain, numbness, and paresthesias of extremities
  - Ataxia of gait, weakness and wasting
  - Loss of deep tendon reflexes
  - Loss of sensation in limbs
  - Impaired vision

- ■ Associated Abnormalities
  - Sensorineural deafness and vertigo
  - Soreness of mucocutaneous junctions of the mouth
  - Stomatoglossitis, corneal degeneration, genital dermatitis

- ■ Treatment
  - Vitamin B and folate supplements

References

Original:
Strachan H. On a form of multiple neuritis prevalent in the West Indies. Practitioner 1897;59:477.

Review and Case Reports:
Roman GC. An epidemic in Cuba of optic neuropathy, sensorineural deafness, peripheral sensory neuropathy and dorsolateral myeloneuropathy. J Neurol Sci 1994 Dec 1;127(1):11–28.
Ropper AH, Samuels MA. Eds: Adams and Victor's Principles of Neurology, 9th ed, New York, McGraw-Hill, 2009. pp1123–4.

Sturge-Weber Syndrome
(alt: Encephalotrigeminal angiomatosis)

- Organs Involved
  - Facial capillaries, cerebral arteries, brain, eyes

- Diagnostic Characteristics
  - Port-wine stain of the face, in trigeminal ophthalmic distribution
  - Ipsilateral leptomeningeal angioma
  - Calcification and atrophy of cerebral cortex

- Associated Abnormalities
  - Seizures
  - Mental retardation
  - Glaucoma in 50 % cases

- Genetics
  - Not inherited. Sporadic occurrence

References

Original:

Sturge WA. A case of partial epilepsy, apparently due to a lesion of one of the vasomotor centres of the brain. Transactions of the Clinical Society of London. 1879;12:162.

Weber FP. Right-sided hemi-hypertrophy resulting from right-sided congenital spastic hemiplegia, with a morbid condition of the left side of the brain, revealed by radiograms. Journal of Neurology and Psychopathology (London). 1922;3:134–139.

Review and Case Reports:

Thomas-Sohl KA, Vaslow DF, Maria BL. Sturge-Weber syndrome: a review. Pediatr Neurol 2004 May;30(5):303–310.

Lo W, Marchuk DA, Ball KL, et al. Brain Vascular Malformation Consortium National Sturge-Weber Syndrome Workgroup. Updates and future horizons on the understanding, diagnosis, and treatment of Sturge-Weber syndrome brain involvement. Dev Med Child Neurol 2012 Mar;54(3):214–223.

SUCLA2 Deficiency Syndrome
(alt: SUCLA2-related mitochondrial DNA depletion syndrome)

- Organs Involved
  - Muscle, spine, basal ganglia, cerebral hemispheres, hearing

- Diagnostic Characteristics
  - Infantile onset hypotonia
  - Severe muscular atrophy
  - Progressive scoliosis or kyphosis
  - Dystonia, athetosis, chorea, hyperkinesia
  - Epilepsy, infantile spasms
  - Growth retardation
  - Severe sensorineural hearing impairment

- Associated Abnormalities
  - Methylmalonic aciduria
  - Elevated plasma methylmalonic acid
  - Elevated plasma lactate
  - Urinary excretion of C4-dicarboxylic-carnitine 20 times normal
  - MRI brain atrophy (mainly putamen and caudate nuclei) and delayed myelination

- Genetics
  - Autosomal recessive inheritance
  - SUCLA2, the only gene associated, involves chromosome 13q14

References

Ostergaard E, Hansen FJ, Sorensen N, et al. Mitochondrial encephalomyopathy with elevated methylmalonic acid is caused by SUCLA2 mutations. Brain 2007;130:853–861.

Carrozzo R, Dionisi-Vici C, Steuerwald U, et al. SUCLA2 mutations are associated with mild methylmalonic aciduria, Leigh-like encephalomyopathy, dystonia and deafness. Brain 2007; 130(3):862–874.

Susac Syndrome
(alt: Retinocochleocerebral vasculopathy)

- Organs Involved
  - Retina, ears, brain, cortical arterioles
- Diagnostic Characteristics
  - Encephalopathy, personality change, headache
  - Multifocal retinal artery occlusions and visual impairment
  - Hearing impairment
  - Female/male ratio 5:1. Age ~30 years
- Associated Abnormalities
  - Multifocal corpus callosal lesions on MRI, resembling vasculitis, and leptomeningeal enhancement
  - Autoimmune disorder
- Differential Diagnosis
- Multiple Sclerosis. ADEM
- Treatment
  - Oral corticosteroids, IV methylprednisolone, or dexamethasone
  - Plasma exchange (PLEX)
  - IV immunoglobulin
  - Cyclophosphamide
- Prognosis
  - Usually self-limiting, but up to 5 years
  - Maybe severe, disabling, and protracted

References

Original:
Susac J, Hardman J, Selhorst J. Microangiopathy of the brain and retina. Neurology 1979;29(3):313.

Review and Case Reports:
Mateen FJ, Zubkov AY, Muralidharan R, et al. Susac syndrome: clinical characteristics and treatment in 29 new cases. Eur J Neurol 2012 Jun;19(6):800–811.

T

Tapia Syndrome – Turner Syndrome

Tapia Syndrome
Terson Syndrome
Thoracic Outlet Syndrome (TOS)
Tolosa-Hunt Syndrome
Tourette Syndrome
Treacher Collins Syndrome
Troyer Syndrome
Turner Syndrome

J.G. Millichap, *Neurological Syndromes: A Clinical Guide to Symptoms and Diagnosis*, DOI 10.1007/978-1-4614-7786-0_19,
© Springer Science+Business Media New York 2013

Tapia Syndrome
(alt: Tapia's vagohypoglossal syndrome; variant of Jackson-MacKenzie syndrome)

- Organs Involved
  - Pharynx, larynx, tongue; cranial nerves X and XII (with or without XI), posterior retroparotid space
- Diagnostic Characteristics
  - Unilateral *para*lysis of pharynx, larynx, and tongue
- Causes
  - Compression injury during transoral intubation in general anesthesia
  - Other injuries to high neck
  - Parotid tumor

References

Original:

Tapia AG. Un caso de paralisis del lado derecho de la laringe y de la lengua, con paralisi del esterno-cleido-mastoidea y trapecio del mismo lado; acompanado de hemiplejia total temporal de lado izquierdo del cuerpo. El Siglo Medico, Madrid 1905;52:211–213.

Tapia AG. Un nouveau syndrome; quelque cas d'hemiplegie dy larynx et de la langue avec ou sans paralysie du sternocleido-mastoidien et du trapeze. Archives internationales de laryngology, d'otologie et de rhinology 1906;22:780–785.

Review and Case Report:

Tesei F, Poveda LM, Strali W, Tosi L, Magnani G, Farneti G. Unilateral laryngeal and hypoglossal paralysis (Tapia's syndrome) following rhinoplasty in general anaesthesia: case report and review of the literature. Acta Otorhinolaryngol Ital 2006 Aug;26(4):219–221.

Terson Syndrome

- Organs Involved
  - Eye, subarachnoid space
- Diagnostic Characteristics
  - Subarachnoid hemorrhage
  - Intraocular hemorrhage (vitreous/subhyaloid)
- Prognosis
  - Higher risk of death

References

Original:
Terson A. De l'hemorrhagie dans le corps vitre au cours de l'hemorrhagie cerebrale. Clin Ophthalmol 1900;6:309–312.
Litten M. Ueber einige vom allgemein klinischen standpunkt aus interessante augenveranderungen. Berl Klin Wochenschr 1881;18:23–27.

Review and Case Reports:
Stienen MN, Lucke S, Gautschi OP, Harders A. Terson haemorrhage in patients suffering aneurysmal subarachnoid haemorrhage: a prospective analysis of 60 consecutive patients. Clin Neurol Neurosurg 2012 Jul;114(6):535–538.

Thoracic Outlet Syndrome (TOS)

- Organs Involved
  - Brachial plexus, subclavian artery, subclavian vein
  - 3 types: neurogenic, arterial, venous TOS
- Diagnostic Characteristics
  - Pain in the hand, arm, shoulder, neck, back
  - Weakness, tingling, decoloration of hand
  - Frozen shoulder
  - Painful, swollen, and blue arm after exercise (Paget-Schroetter syndrome)
- Causes
  - Trauma, injury from car accident, a job, use of computer, sports related
  - Extra rib causing compression on plexus or artery (cervical rib syndrome)
  - Compression by muscle (scalenus anticus syndrome)
  - Narrowing between clavicle and first rib (costoclavicular syndrome)
  - Pancoast tumor, a rare cause
- Tests
  - "Stick em up hand raise:" affected hand is paler when raised above head.
  - "Compression test:" pressure between clavicle and humeral head causes pain and numbness in affected arm.
  - Electrophysiological.
  - MRI/MRI of brachial plexus.
- Treatment
  - Stretching and/or physical therapy
  - Postural exercises
  - Cortisone injections, botox
  - Surgery when noninvasive approach fails

References

Reviews and Case Reports:

Pang D, Wessel HB. Thoracic outlet syndrome. Neurosurg 1988 Jan;22(1 Pt 1):105–121.

Christo PJ, McGreevy K. Updated perspectives on neurogenic thoracic outlet syndrome. Curr Pain Headache Rep 2011 Feb;15(1):14–21.

Tubbs RS, Muhleman M, Miller J, et al. Cervical ribs with neurological sequelae in children: a case series. Childs Nerv Syst 2012 Apr;28(4):605–608.

Ferrante MA. The thoracic outlet syndromes. Muscle Nerve 2012 Jun;45(6):780–795.

Tolosa-Hunt Syndrome

- Organs Involved
  - Cavernous sinus, eyes; cranial nerves III, IV, V, VI; extraocular muscles

- Diagnostic Characteristics
  - Unilateral, recurrent, sharp retro-orbital headache
  - Extraocular III, IV, V, VI palsies
  - MRI or biopsy documentation of granuloma and inflammation

- Associated Abnormalities
  - Ipsilateral proptosis
  - Sensory loss over forehead
  - Sluggish pupil reaction to light
  - Blurred vision

- Cause
  - Granulomatous infiltration with inflammation or tumor in the cavernous sinus or superior orbital fissure

- Differential Diagnosis
  - Craniopharyngioma. Meningioma
  - Migraine

- Treatment
  - Corticosteroids. Immunosuppressive agents

- Prognosis
  - Usually good. Spontaneous remission may occur
  - Relapse in ~30–40 % patients

References

Original:

Tolosa E. Periarteritic lesions of carotid siphon with clinical features of a carotid infraclinoid aneurysm. J Neurol, Neurosurg and Psychiatry, London. 1954;17:300–302.

Tolosa E, Fuenmayor P, Llovet J. Syndrome du sinus caverneux. Considerations sur ses formes benignes et spontanement regressives. Revue d'oto-neuro-ophthamologie, Paris. 1961;33:365–368.

Hunt WE, Meagher JN, LeFever HE, Zeman W. Painful ophthalmoplegia. Its relation to indolent inflammation of the cavernous sinus. Neurology 1961;11:56–62.

Review and Case Reports:

La Mantia L, Curone C, Rapoport AM, Bussone G: International Headache Society. Cephalalgia 2006 Jul;26(7):772–781.

Colnaghi S, Versino M, Marchioni E, et al. ICHD-II diagnostic criteria for Tolosa-Hunt syndrome in idiopathic inflammatory syndromes of the orbit and/or the cavernous sinus. Cephalalgia 2008 Jun;28(6):577–584.

Tourette Syndrome

- Organs Involved
  - Eyes, face, shoulders, neck, larynx
- Diagnostic Characteristics
  - Chronic tics, motor and vocal, persisting for longer than 1 year
- Definition and Differential Diagnosis
  - Chronic tic disorder is manifested by either motor or vocal tics, occurring intermittently for more than 1 year.
  - Transient tic disorder lasts for at least 2 weeks, but no longer than 1 year.
  - Tic or habit spasm is an involuntary, recurrent twitch or motor movement (motor tic) or a grunt or vocalization (vocal tic).
  - Simple motor tics involve the eyes (blepharospasm), the face (grimacing) and the head, neck, and shoulders (jerking, twisting, and shrugging movements).
  - Simple vocal tics include throat clearing, grunting, sniffing, and barking.
  - Complex motor tics are gestures, jumping, and touching objects.
  - Complex vocal tics are utterances of obscene language (coprolalia); repeated words or phrases, sometimes out of context (palilalia); and repeated words said by another person (echolalia).
  - Maybe precipitated by a physical or emotional stimulus, controlled partially by will; tics are infrequent during sleep, exaggerated by stress and fatigue, and lessened by diverting attention.
- Genetics
  - Autosomal dominant mode of inheritance
  - Environmental factors in addition to genetics play a role in causation

References

Original:
George Gilles de la Tourette described the syndrome in 1885 (English translation by Lajonchere C, et al. Historical review of Gilles de la Tourette syndrome. Arch Neurol 1996;53:567–574.)

Review and Case Reports:
Eapen V, Moriarty J, Robertson MM. Stimulus induced behaviors in Tourette's syndrome. J Neurol Neurosurg Psychiatry. 1994;57:853–855.
Knight T, Steeves T, Day L, Lowerison M, Jette N, Pringsheim T. Prevalence of tic disorders: a systematic review and meta-analysis. Pediatr Neurol 2012 Aug;47(2):77–90.

Treacher Collins Syndrome
(alt: Treacher Collins-Franceschetti syndrome; mandibulofacial dysostosis)

- Organs Involved
  - Head, face, ears, facial nerve, eyes, palate, and airway

- Diagnostic Characteristics
  - Underdeveloped mandible and zygoma of face
  - Ear anomalies: small or absent ears, atresia of external auditory canals, dysmorphic ossicles and middle ear, conductive hearing loss
  - Facial nerve of the mastoid portion displaced more lateral and anterior
  - Eye abnormalities: coloboma, downslanting palpebral fissures, absent eyelashes
  - Cleft palate
  - Airway problems, result of mandibular hypoplasia

- Associated Abnormalities
  - Dental anomalies
  - Ocular hypertelorism
  - Choanal atresia
  - Macrostomia

- Genetics
  - Autosomal dominant inheritance
  - Mutations in the TCOF1 gene

- Prognosis
  - Mentality usually normal.
  - Constricted airway is a life-threatening problem during anesthesia.
  - Facial deformity may affect quality of life.

References

Original:
Treacher Collin E. Cases with symmetrical congenital notches in the outer part of each lid and defective development of the malar bones. Trans Ophthalmol Soc UK 1900;20:190–192.
Franceschetti A, Klein D. Mandibulo-facial dysostosis: new hereditary syndrome. Acta Ophthalmol 1949;27:143–224.

Reviews and Case Reports:
Gorlin RJ. Syndromes of the Head and Neck. Oxford University Press, 2001, 4th edition.
Takegoshi H, Kaga K, Kikuchi S, Ito K. Mandibulofacial dysostosis: CT evaluation of the temporal bones for surgical risk assessment in patients of bilateral aural atresia. Int J Pediatr Otorhinolaryngol 2000 Aug 11;54(1):33–40.
Duggan M, Ames W, Papsin B, Berdock S. Facial nerve palsy: a complication following anaesthesia in a child with Treacher Collins syndrome. Paediatr Anaesth 2004 Jul;14(7):604–606.
Luquetti DV, Hing AV, Rieder MJ, et al. "Mandibulofacial dysostosis with microcephaly" caused by EFTUD2 mutations: Expanding the phenotype. Am J Med Genet A 2012 Dec 14; [Epub ahead of print].

Troyer Syndrome
(alt: Cross-McKusick syndrome; SPG20)

- Organs Involved
  - Brain, muscles
- Diagnostic Characteristics
  - Distal amyotrophy: muscle wasting, with onset in childhood, affecting thenar, hypothenar, and dorsal interosseous muscles
  - Spasticity and contractures of lower limbs, ankle clonus
  - Dysarthria, drooling, mild cerebellar dysmetria
  - Mild choreoathetosis
  - Mental retardation
- Associated Abnormalities
  - Hammer toes, pes cavus, short stature
  - Kyphoscoliosis
  - Emotional liability
- Genetics
  - Autosomal recessive inheritance.
  - Mutations in SPG20 gene that encodes the protein spartin, especially frequent in the Amish and Omani populations.
  - Troyer is the Amish family in which the syndrome was first described.

References

Original:
Cross HE, McKusick VA. The Troyer syndrome: a recessive form of spastic paraplegia with distal muscle wasting. Arch Neurol 1967;16:473–485.

Review and Case Reports:
Auer-Grumbach M, Fazekas F, Radner H, et al. Troyer syndrome: a combination of central brain abnormality and motor neuron disease? J Neurol 1999;246(7):556–561.
Proukakis C, Cross H, Patel H, et al. Troyer syndrome revisited. A clinical and radiological study of a complicated hereditary spastic paraplegia. J Neurol 2004 Sp;251(9):1105–1110.

Turner Syndrome
(alt: Ullrich-Turner syndrome; gonadal dysgenesis)

- ■ Organs Involved
  - • Chest, face, neck, ears, heart, kidneys, gonads, brain

- ■ Diagnostic Characteristics
  - • Short stature
  - • Lymphedema of hands and feet
  - • Broad (shield) chest
  - • Webbed neck
  - • Amenorrhea, underdeveloped ovaries and breasts (gonadal dysfunction)
  - • Obesity, type 2 diabetes, hypertension, hypothyroidism in adulthood

- ■ Associated Abnormalities
  - • Coarctation of the aorta
  - • Horseshoe kidney
  - • Hearing impairment
  - • ADHD
  - • Nonverbal learning disability (math, visuospatial perception deficits)

- ■ Genetics
  - • Single X chromosome (45,X) monosomy or mosaicism

References

Original:
Turner HH. A syndrome of infantilism, congenital webbed neck, and cubitus valgus. Endocrinology 1938;23:566–574.

Review and Case Reports:
Hong DS, Reiss AL. Cognition and Behavior in Turner syndrome: a brief review. Pediatr Endocrinol Rev 2012 May;9 Suppl 2:710–712.
Trolle C, Mortensen KH, Hjerrild BE, Cleemann L, Gravholt CH. Clinical care of adult Turner syndrome – new aspects. Pediatr Endocrinol Rev 2012 May;9 Suppl 2:739–749.

U

Usher Syndrome Type 1

Usher Syndrome Type 1

J.G. Millichap, *Neurological Syndromes: A Clinical Guide to Symptoms and Diagnosis*, DOI 10.1007/978-1-4614-7786-0_20,
© Springer Science+Business Media New York 2013

Usher Syndrome Type 1
(alt: Hallgren syndrome; Usher-Hallgren syndrome; retinitis pigmentosa-dysacusis syndrome)

- Organs Involved
  - Inner ear, retina
- Diagnostic Characteristics
  - Sensorineural hearing loss, congenital
  - Visual impairment, early night blindness, tunnel vision
  - Adolescent onset of retinitis pigmentosa, with constricted visual fields
  - Leading cause of deafblindness
- Associated Abnormalities
  - Vestibular problems
  - Slow to develop walking
  - Speech impairment, unless fitted with cochlear implant
- Genetics
  - Autosomal recessive inheritance
  - Mutations in one of several different genes, including USH1G
- Differential Diagnosis
  - Type II Usher syndrome, milder form with hard-of-hearing and normal vestibular system; mutations in one of three different genes: USH2A, GPR98, and DFNB31
  - Type III Usher syndrome, progressive loss of hearing, vision, and vestibular dysfunction; Finnish population most susceptible; mutations in CLRN1 gene

References

Original:
Usher C. On the inheritance of retinitis pigmentosa with notes of cases. Roy Lond Ophthalmol Hosp Rep 1914;19:130–236.
Von Grafe A. Exceptionelles verhalten des gesichtsfeldes bei pigmententartung der netzhaut. Archiv fur Ophthalmologie 1858;4:250–253.

Review and Case Reports:
Henricson C, Wass M, Lidestam B, Moller C, Lyxell B. Cognitive skills in children with Usher syndrome type 1 and cochlear implants. Int J Pediatr Otorhinolaryngol 2012 Oct;76(10): 1449–1457.

V

Velo-Cardio-Facial Syndrome – Vogt-Koyanagi-Harada Syndrome

Velo-Cardio-Facial Syndrome
Verbiest Syndrome
Verger-Dejerine Syndrome
Vernet Syndrome
Vici Syndrome
Villaret Syndrome
Vogt-Koyanagi-Harada Syndrome

J.G. Millichap, *Neurological Syndromes: A Clinical Guide to Symptoms and Diagnosis*, DOI 10.1007/978-1-4614-7786-0_21,
© Springer Science+Business Media New York 2013

Velo-Cardio-Facial Syndrome
(alt: DiGeorge syndrome, 22q11.2 deletion syndrome)

- Organs Involved
  - Palate, heart, face, nervous system, renal, parathyroid

- Diagnostic Characteristics of CATCH-22
  - C: Cardiac abnormality (tetralogy of Fallot)
  - A: Abnormal facies (hypertelorism)
  - T: Thymic aplasia
  - C: Cleft palate
  - H: Hypocalcemia/hypoparathyroidism
  - 22-Chromosome abnormality

- Associated Abnormalities
  - Learning and expressive language deficits (90 %)
  - Speech hypernasality, delayed vocabulary acquisition, and dysarthria
  - Specific neuropsychological profile, borderline IQ
  - Schizophrenia
  - Seizures (with or without hypocalcemia)
  - Hearing loss (conductive and sensorineural)
  - Basal ganglia and periventricular calcification
  - Autoimmune disorders

- Genetics
  - De novo deletions on chromosome 22q11.2
  - One in two chance of passing deletion 22q to offspring
  - Autosomal recessive or X-linked traits

- Treatment
  - Identify immune problems and treat early
  - Cardiac surgery often required
  - Vitamin D and calcium for hypoparathyroidism
  - Neuropsychological testing and IEP (individual education program)

References

Original:
DiGeorge AM. Congenital absence of the thymus and its immunologic consequences: concurrence with congenital hypoparathyroidism. White Plains, NY: March of Dimes-Birth Defects Foundation. 1968;IV(1):116–121.

Review and Case Report:
Kinoshita H, Kokudo T, Ide T, et al. A patient with DiGeorge syndrome with spina bifida and sacral myelomeningocele who developed both hypocalcemia-induced seizure and epilepsy. Seizure 2010 Jun;19(5):303–305.
Robin NH, Shprintzen RJ. Defining the clinical spectrum of deletion 22q11.2. J Pediatr 2005; 147(1):90–96.

Verbiest Syndrome
(alt: Lumbar spinal stenosis)

- Organs Involved
  - Lumbar vertebral canal, cauda equina
- Diagnostic Characteristics
  - Narrowing of the lumbar vertebral canal in middle-aged and older men
  - Symptoms of compression of caudal nerve roots on standing or walking but not at rest
- Prognosis
  - Progressive
- Treatment
  - Conservative (physiotherapy) or/and surgical

References

Original:
Verbiest H. A radicular syndrome from developmental narrowing of the lumbar vertebral canal. J Bone Joint Surg Br 1954 May;36-B(2):230–237.

Review and Case Reports:
Storm PB, Chou D, Tamargo RJ. Lumbar spinal stenosis, cauda equina syndrome, and multiple lumbosacral radiculopathies. Phys Med Rehabil Clin N Am 2002;13:713–733.

Verger-Dejerine Syndrome
(alt: Anterior parietal lobe syndrome)

- Organs Involved
  - Parietal lobe
- Diagnostic Characteristics
  - Inability to discriminate sensory functions of the opposite side of the body
  - Loss of position sense and sense of movement and distance
  - Inability to localize touch and pain stimuli
  - Astereognosis

References

Original:
Verger H. In: Progress medical, Paris.1910:519.
Dejerine J, Manson J. Un nouveau type de syndrome sensitive corticale observe dans un cas de monoplegic corticale dissocie. Revue neurologique, Paris. 1914–1915;28:1265.
Holmes GM. Disturbances of visual orientation. Brit J Ophthalmology, London 1918;2:449–468, 506–516.

Review and Case Reports:
Ropper AH, Samuels MA. Eds Adams and Victor's Principals of Neurology, ninth edition. New York, McGraw Hill, 2009.

Vernet Syndrome
(alt: Collet-Sicard syndrome; Jugular foramen syndrome)

- Organs Involved
  - Cranial nerves IX, X, XI (and XII), jugular foramen
- Diagnostic Characteristics
  - Hoarse voice, dysarthria
  - Deviation of uvula to normal side
  - Dysphagia
  - Loss of taste sensation posterior 1/3 of tongue
  - Decrease parotid gland secretion
  - Absent gag reflex
  - Paralysis of sternocleidomastoid and trapezius muscles
  - When XII cranial nerve also involved, referred to as Collet-Sicard syndrome
- Causes
  - Jugular foramen involved by:
  - Tumor (glomus, meningioma, acoustic neuroma, metastatic)
  - Aneurysm
  - Trauma
  - Infection

References

Schweinfurth JM, Johnson JT, Weissman J. Jugular foramen syndrome as a complication of metastatic melanoma. Am J Otolaryngol 1993 May-Jun;14(3):168–174.

Kawabe K, Sekine T, Murata K, et al. A case of Vernet syndrome with varicella zoster virus infection. J Neurol Sci 2008 Jul 15;270(1–2):209–210.

Hashimoto T, Watanabe O, Takase M, Koniyama J, Kobota M. Collet-Sicard syndrome after minor head trauma. Neurosurgery 1988 Sep;23(3):367–370.

V Velo-Cardio-Facial Syndrome – Vogt-Koyanagi-Harada Syndrome

Vici Syndrome
(alt: Immunodeficiency with cataract, hypopigmentation and absent corpus callosum)

- Organs Involved
  - Skin, brain, eyes, face
- Diagnostic Characteristics
  - Agenesis of corpus callosum
  - Hypotonia
  - Developmental delay
  - Albinism
  - Cataracts
  - Immunodeficiency, recurrent infection
- Associated Abnormalities
  - Cardiomyopathy
  - Nystagmus, optic nerve atrophy
  - Seizures
  - Psychomotor retardation
  - Sensorineural hearing loss
- Genetics
  - Autosomal recessive inheritance
  - Cause unknown
- Prognosis
  - Poor because of recurrent severe infection and immunodeficiency

References

Original:
Vici CD, Sabetta G, Gambarara M, et al. Agenesis of the corpus callosum, combined immunodeficiency, bilateral cataract, and hypopigmentation in two brothers. Am J Med Genet 1988;29(1):1–8.

Review and Case Report:
Ozkale M, Erol I, Gumus A, Ozkale Y, Alehan F. Vici syndrome associated with sensorineural hearing loss and laryngomalacia. Pediatr Neurol 2012 Nov;47:375–378.

Villaret Syndrome

- ■ Organs Involved
  - • IX, X, XI, XII cranial nerves and cervical sympathetic ganglia, posterior retroparotid space
- ■ Diagnostic Characteristics
  - • IX nerve paralysis – loss of taste posterior third of tongue
  - • X paralysis – loss of sensation soft palate, pharynx, larynx
  - • XI paralysis – sternocleidomastoid and trapezius
  - • XII paralysis – ispsilateral deviation of tongue
  - • Sympathetic involvement – Horner's syndrome
  - • Lesion in posterior retroparotid space
- ■ Causes
  - • Tumors of parotid gland, carotid body, lymph nodes, tuberculous adenitis, sarcoid, fungal lesions, carotid artery dissection

References

Original:
Villaret M. Le syndrome nerveux de l'espace retro-porotidien posterieur. Revue neurologique, Paris 1916;23(1):188–190.

Review and Case Report:
Szulc-Kuberska J, Klimek A, Hajdukiewicz Z, Radomska M. Case of Collet-Sicard-Villaret syndrome caused by metastasis of renal carcinoma. Neurol Neurochir Pol 1978;12(5):659–661.

Vogt-Koyanagi-Harada Syndrome
(alt: VKH syndrome, uveodermatologic syndrome)

- Organs Involved
  - Melanocyte-containing organs, eye, hair, skin, meninges
- Diagnostic Characteristics
  - Uveitis
  - Poliosis
  - Vitiligo
  - Aseptic meningoencephalitis
  - Loss of pigment and hair on eyelids, nose, and lips
  - Headache, deafness, vertigo
- Differential Diagnosis
  - Viral meningoencephalitis
- Treatment
  - Immunosuppressive drugs, prednisone and azathioprine
- Prognosis
  - Guarded

References

Original:
Vogt A. Fruhzeitiges ergrauen der zilien und bemerkungen uber den sogenannten plutzlichen eintritt dieser veranderung. Klinische Monatsblatter fur Augenheilkunde, Stuttgart. 1906;44: 228–242.
Koyanagi Y. Dysakusis, alopecia and poliosis bei schwerer uveitis nicht traumatischen ursprungs. Klinische Monatsblatter fur Augenheilkunde, Stuttgart. 1929;82:194–211.
Harada E. Clinical study of nonsuppurative choroiditis. A report of acute diffuse choroiditis. Acta Societatis ophthalmologicae Japonicae. 1926;30:356.

Review and Case Reports:
Tahara T, Sekitani T. Neurological evaluation of Harada's disease. Acta Otolaryngol Suppl 1995;519:110–113.
Kamondi A, Szegedi A, Papp A, Seres A, Szirmai I. Vogt-Koyanagi-Harada disease presenting initially as aseptic meningoencephalitis. Eur J Neurol 2000 Nov;7(6): 719–722.
Loh Y. Basilar leptomeningitis in Vogt-Koyanagi-Harada disease. Neurology 2012 Feb 7;78(6): 438–439.
Smit J, Berman DC, Nielsen H. Vogt-Koyanagi-Harada syndrome: a rare but important differential diagnosis of viral meningitis. Scand J Infect Dis 2012 Feb;44(2):157–159.

W

Walker-Warburg Syndrome – Wolfram Syndrome

Walker-Warburg Syndrome
Wallenberg Syndrome
Wartenberg Syndrome
Weber Syndrome
Werdnig-Hoffman Syndrome
Wernicke-Korsakoff Syndrome
West Syndrome
Williams Syndrome
Wolf-Hirschhorn Syndrome
Wolfram Syndrome

J.G. Millichap, *Neurological Syndromes: A Clinical Guide to Symptoms and Diagnosis*, DOI 10.1007/978-1-4614-7786-0_22,

Walker-Warburg Syndrome
(alt: Chemke syndrome; HARD syndrome [hydrocephalus, agyria, retinal dysplasia]; Pagon syndrome; cerebro-ocular dysplasia-muscular dystrophy syndrome)

- Organs Involved
  - Brain, muscles, eyes

- Diagnostic Characteristics
  - Lissencephaly
  - Hydrocephalus
  - Cerebellar malformations
  - Eye abnormalities (retinal dysplasia)
  - Congenital muscular dystrophy, a dystroglycanopathy

- Associated Abnormalities
  - Congenital hypotonia
  - Developmental delay
  - Mental retardation
  - Seizures

- Genetics
  - Autosomal recessive inheritance
  - Mutations in several genes, POMT1, POMT2, FKTN, FKRP, ISPD
  - One-third cases unexplained

- Prognosis
  - Poor. Most die before age 3 years

References

Original:
Walker AE. Lissencephaly. Arch Neurol & Psychiatry (Chicago) 1942;48:13–29.
Warburg M. The heterogeneity of microphthalmia in the mentally retarded. Birth Defects Orig Arctic Ser 1971 Mar;7(3):136–154.

Review and Case Reports:
Devisme L, Bouchet C, Gonzales M, et al. Cobblestone lissencephaly: neuropathological subtypes and correlations with genes of dystroglycanopathies. Brain 2012 Feb;135(Pt 2):469–482.

Wallenberg Syndrome
(alt: Lateral medullary syndrome (LMS); posterior-inferior cerebellar artery syndrome (PICA))

- Organs Involved
  - Medulla, vertebral, and posterior inferior cerebellar arteries (PICA)

- Diagnostic characteristics   Dysfunction
  Ipsilateral:

Diagnostic characteristics	Dysfunction
Loss of facial pain/temperature sensation	Spinal V nucleus/tract
Decreased taste	Tractus solitarius
Dysphonia, dysphagia	Nucleus ambiguous X
Paralysis of palate, vocal cord, pharynx	Nucleus ambiguous X
Ataxia/dysmetria	Inferior cerebellar peduncle
Horner's syndrome	Descending sympathetic

  Contralateral:

Loss of body pain/temperature sensation	Lateral spinothalamic tract
Vertigo, vomiting, nystagmus	Vestibular nuclei

- Associated Abnormalities
  - Constant hiccups
  - Chronic neuropathic pain

- Cause
  - Infarct/occlusion of PICA or vertebral artery

- Treatment
  - Stroke rehabilitation regimen
  - Feeding tube or gastrostomy
  - Gabapentin for pain
  - Aspirin

- Prognosis
  - Mostly good. Ataxia is the commonest sequel.

References

Original:
Wallenberg A. Acute bulbaraffection (Embolle der arteria cerebelli posterior inferior sinistra). Archiv fur Psychiatrie und Nervenkrankheiten, Berlin. 1895;27:504–540.

Review and Case Reports:
Riqueiro-Veloso MT, Pego-Reigosa R, Branas-Fernandez F, Martinez-Vazquez F, Cortes-Laino JA. Wallenberg syndrome: a review of 25 cases. Rev Neurol 1997 Oct;25(146):1561–1564.

Wartenberg Syndrome
(alt: Handcuff neuropathy; wristlet-watch syndrome; cheiralgia paresthetica)

- Organs Involved
  - Superficial branch of the radial nerve
- Diagnostic Characteristics
  - Numbness, tingling, and weakness of lateral aspect of thumb and wrist
  - Tinel's sign positive over radial styloid process
- Differential Diagnosis
  - Wartenberg's migratory sensory neuropathy
  - Wallenberg syndrome (lateral medullary syndrome)
- Treatment
  - Conservative: removal of tight watch strap, splint

References

Original:
Wartenberg R. Cheiralgia paraesthetica. Zeitschrift fur die gesamte Neurologie und Psychiatrie 1932;141:145–155.

Review and Case Reports:
Braidwood AS. Superficial radial neuropathy. J Bone and Joint Surg 1975;57-B(3):380–383.
Lanzetta M, Foucher G. Entrapment of the superficial branch of the radial nerve (Wartenberg's syndrome): a report of 52 cases. International Orthopaedics 1993 Dec;17(6):342–345.
Tosun N, Tuncay I, Akpinar F. Entrapment of the sensory branch of the radial nerve (Wartenberg's syndrome): an unusual case. Tohoku J Exp Med 2001 Mar;193(3):251–254.

Weber Syndrome

- Organs Involved
  - Ventral midbrain, oculomotor nerve, cerebral peduncle, contralateral limbs
- Diagnostic Characteristics
  - Ipsilateral ptosis, dilated pupil, exotropia, diplopia (CN III palsy)
  - Contralateral (crossed) hemiparesis (corticospinal tract involved)
  - Contralateral parkinsonism (substantia nigra involved)
- Cause
  - Midbrain infarction result of occlusion of paramedian branches of posterior cerebral artery or basilar perforating arteries
  - Aneurysm
  - Neoplasm in pituitary region maybe associated

References

Original:
Weber HD. A contribution to the pathology of the crura cerebri. Medico-Chirurgical Transactions, London. 1863;46:121–139.
Grasset J. Un type special de paralysie alterne motrice etc. Revue Neurologique, Paris. 1900;8:586.
Gubler AM. Gazette hebdomadaire de medicine et de chjirurgie, Paris. 1856;3:749–754.
(English translation in Wolf. The Classical Brain Stem Syndromes. Springfield, IL, Thomas, 1971)

Reviews:
Silverman IE, Liu GT, Volpe NJ, Galetta SL. The crossed paralyses. The original brain-stem syndromes of Millard-Gubler, Foville, Weber, and Raymond-Cestan. Arch Neurol 1995 Jun; 52(6):635–638.
Schmidt D. Classical brain stem syndrome. Definitions and history. Ophthalmologe 2000 Jun;97(6):411–417.

Werdnig-Hoffman Syndrome
(alt: Spinal muscular atrophy type 1)

- Organs Involved
  - Muscles, spinal anterior horn cells, and bulbar motor neurons
- Diagnostic Characteristics
  - Infantile onset, 0–6 months, "floppy infant syndrome" SMA type 1.
  - Proximal muscles are first affected and followed by flaccid quadriplegia.
  - Tongue fasciculations.
  - Absent reflexes.
  - Extraocular muscles are spared.
  - Majority (~85 %) die by age 2 years.
- Differential Diagnosis
  - SMA type 2, onset age 6 months to 1 year, survival past age 2 years
  - SMA type 3 (Kugelberg-Welander disease), onset late childhood
  - Fazio-Londe syndrome (childhood bulbar muscular atrophy)
  - Congenital muscular dystrophy
  - Limp infant syndrome, various causes
- Genetics
  - Autosomal recessive inheritance, deletion or mutation in SMN1 gene

References

Original:
Werdnig G. Zwei frühinfantile hereditäre Fälle von progressiver Muskelatrophie unter dem Bilde der Dystrophie, aber auf neurotischer Grundlage. Archiv für Psychiatrie und Nervenkrankheiten, Berlin. 1891; 22: 437–481.
Hoffmann J. Weitere Beiträge zur Lehre von der progressiven neurotischen Muskeldystrophie. Deutsche Zeitschrift für Nervenheilkunde, Berlin. 1891;1: 95–120.

Reviews and Case Reports:
Wadman RI, Bosboom WM, van der Pol WL, et al. Drug treatment for spinal muscular atrophy type 1. Cochrane Database Syst Rev 2012 Apr18;4:CD006281.
Sproule DM, Hasnain R, Koenigsberger D, Montgomery M, De Vivo DC, Kaufmann P. Age at disease onset predicts likelihood and rapidity of growth failure among infants and young children with spinal muscular atrophy types 1 and 2. J Child Neurol 2012 Jul;27(7):845–851.

Wernicke-Korsakoff Syndrome
(alt: Korsakoff psychosis; Wernicke encephalopathy; wet brain)

- Organs Involved
  - Mamillary bodies of brain, thalamus, basal forebrain, median and dorsal raphe nuclei, cerebellum

- Diagnostic Characteristics

- Wernicke encephalopathy:
  - Confusion
  - Nystagmus, ophthalmoplegia, anisocoria, sluggish pupils
  - Ataxia
  - Coma and death if untreated

- Korsakoff psychosis:
  - Amnesia, anterograde and retrograde
  - Confabulation
  - Hallucinations
  - Dislike of sunlight

- Causes and Pathology
  - Acute thiamine deficiency in Wernicke encephalopathy.
  - Korsakoff psychosis is a chronic neurologic sequela after Wernicke encephalopathy.
  - Malnourished chronic alcoholics are susceptible.
  - Prolonged IV therapy without vitamin B1 supplementation.
  - Diets consisting mainly of polished rice (thiamine deficient).
  - Glucose loading plus deficient thiamine precipitates onset of overt encephalopathy (thiamine pyrophosphate is a glucose metabolism cofactor).
  - Cytotoxic edema of brain and degeneration of mamillary bodies are important in memory circuits (e.g., Papez circuit).
  - Degeneration of medial thalami, tectum, and periaqueductal areas.

- Treatment
  - Supplemental thiamine IV followed by oral doses.
  - Glucose infusions delayed until thiamine deficiency is corrected, since encephalopathy may worsen in absence of thiamine.
  - Complete recovery unlikely if amnesia and psychosis have developed.

References

Original:

Wernicke K. Die acute, hamorrhagische polioencephalitis superior. In: Lehrbuch der Gehirnkrankheiten; Kassel, Fischer, and Berlin 1881;22:229–242.

Korsakoff SS. Ob alkogol'nom paraliche. Westnick Psychiatrii, Moscow 1887 vol 4. Uber eine besondere form psychiser storung kombiniert mit multipler neuritis. Archiv fur Psychiatrie und Nervenkrankheiten, Berlin 1890;21:669–704.

West Syndrome

- Organs Involved
  - Brain
- Diagnostic Characteristics
  - Infantile spasms
  - Hypsarrhythmia
  - Developmental delay
- Etiology
  - Known in ~60 % and unidentified in ~40 %; genetic factors in some
  - Etiologies prenatal (~50 %), perinatal (33 %), postnatal (6 %)
  - Hypoxic-ischemic-encephalopathy (10 %)
  - Chromosomal abnormalities (8 %), malformations (8 %), stroke (8 %)
  - Tuberous sclerosis complex (7 %), periventricular leukomalacia (5 %)
- Treatment
  - ACTH, corticosteroids
  - Vigabatrin, especially those with tuberous sclerosis
  - Ketogenic diet
- Prognosis
  - Generally poor, high proportion (~90 %) with psychomotor retardation.
  - Idiopathic cases do better than those with known etiology.
  - Prompt diagnosis and treatment may improve response.

References

Original:

West WJ. On a peculiar form of infantile convulsions. Letter. Lancet 1840–41;1:724–725.

Gibbs FA, Gibbs EL. Hypsarrhythmia. Atlas of Electroencephalography, vol 2. Reading, MA; Addison-Wesley, 1952.

Review and Case Reports:

Millichap JG, Bickford RG, Klass DW, Backus RE. Infantile spasms, hypsarrhythmia, and mental retardation. A study of etiologic factors in 61 patients. Epilepsia 1962;3:188.

Millichap JG, Bickford. Infantile spasms, hypsarrhythmia, and mental retardation. Response to corticotrophin and its relation to age and etiology in 21 patients. JAMA 1962;182:523.

Osborne JP, Lux AL, Edwards SW, et al. The underlying etiology of infantile spasms (West syndrome): information from the United Kingdom Infantile Spasms Study (UKISS) on contemporary causes and their classification. Epilepsia 2010 Oct;51(10):2168–2174.

Paciorkowski AR, Thio LL, Dobyns WB. Genetic and biologic classification of infantile spasms. Pediatr Neurol 2011 Dec;45(6):355–367.

W   Walker-Warburg Syndrome – Wolfram Syndrome

Williams Syndrome

- Organs Involved
  - Face, heart, nervous system, blood calcium
- Diagnostic Characteristics
  - "Elfin" facial appearance, puffy eyes, long philtrum
  - Supravalvular aortic stenosis
  - Developmental delay, language delay, borderline IQ or below
  - Highly verbal, overly sociable, "cocktail party" personality type
  - Fondness for music
  - Visual spatial deficits
  - Failure to thrive
  - Elevated serum calcium
- Associated Abnormalities
  - Structural deficits of cerebellum, right parietal, and left frontal cortex
  - Ataxia, hyperreflexia, nystagmus
  - ADHD
- Genetics
  - Deletion of ~26 genes on region of q11.23 of chromosome 7

References

Original:

Williams JC, Barratt-Boyes BG, Lowe JB. Supravalvular aortic stenosis. Circulation 1961;24:1311–1318.

Beuren AJ, Apitz J, Harmjanz D. Supravalvular aortic stenosis in association with mental retardation and a certain facial appearance. Circulation 1962;26:1235–1240.

Review and Case Reports:

Bellugi U, Bihrle A, Jernigan T, Trauner D, Doherty S. Neuropsychological, neurological, and neuroanatomical profile of Williams syndrome. Am J Med Genet Suppl 1990;6:115–125.

Wolf-Hirschhorn Syndrome

- Organs Involved
  - Head, face, brain, muscle, heart
- Diagnostic Characteristics
  - Craniofacial phenotype (microcephaly, micrognathia, short philtrum, hypertelorism, dysplastic ears, and tags)
  - Mental and growth retardation
  - Muscle hypotonia
  - Seizures (50–100 % cases)
  - Skeletal anomalies (60–70 %)
  - Congenital heart defects
- Associated Less Common Abnormalities
  - Structural brain anomalies (33 %)
  - Hypospadias, renal anomalies
  - Coloboma of iris
  - Deafness
  - Immunodeficiency and IgA deficiency
- Genetics
  - Partial deletion of short arm of chromosome 4 at 4p16.3
  - De novo deletion in ~87 % cases, 80 % paternally derived
  - From parent with chromosome translocation in ~13 %, 2/1 maternal/ paternal transmission

References

Original:
Cooper H, Hirschhorn K. Apparent deletion of short arms of one chromosome (4 or 5) in a child with defects of midline fusion. Mammalian Chrom Nwsl 1961;4:14.
Hirschhorn K, Cooper HL, Firschein IL. Deletion of short arms of chromosome 4–5 in a child with defects of midline fusion. Humangenetik 1965;1(5):479–482.
Wolf U, Reinwein H, Porsch R, Schroter R, Baitsch H. Deficiency on the short arms of a chromosome No.4. Humangenetik 1965;1(5):397–413.

Review and Case Reports:
Hammond P, Hannes F, Suttie M, et al. Fine-grained facial phenotype-genotype analysis in Wolf-Hirschhorn syndrome. Eur J Hum Genet 2012 Jan;20(1):33–40.
Fisch GS, Grossfeld P, Falk R, Battaglia A, Youngblom J, Simensen R. Cognitive-behavioral features of Wolf-Hirschhorn syndrome and other subtelomeric microdeletions. Am J Med Genet C Semin Med Genet 2010 Nov 15;154C(4):417–426.
Battaglia A, Carey JC, South ST, Wright TJ. Wolf-Hirschhorn syndrome. In: Pagon RA, Bird TD, Dolan CR, et al., editors. GeneReviews [internet], Seattle (WA): University of Washington, Seattle, 1993- Update June 17, 2010.

Wolfram Syndrome
(alt: DIDMOAD)

- Organs Involved
  - Pancreas, optic nerve, inner ear, brainstem, mitochondria
- Diagnostic Characteristics
  - *Di*abetes *i*nsipidus, *di*abetes *m*ellitus
  - *O*ptic *a*trophy
  - *D*eafness
- Associated Abnormalities
  - Neurological manifestations: dysarthria, seizures, anosmia, nystagmus, ataxia
  - Brainstem and cerebellar atrophy on CT scan and NMR
  - Manifestations of olivopontocerebellar atrophy
- Genetics
  - Mutations in WFS1, the wolframin gene, are located on the long arm of chromosome 4, the 4p16.1 region.
  - Loss of wolframin disrupts the production of insulin, causing diabetes, and possibly calcium homeostasis.
  - Inheritance is autosomal recessive, dominant, or mitochondrial.

References

Original:
Wolfram DJ, Wagener HP. Diabetes mellitus and simple optic atrophy among siblings: report of four cases. Mayo Clin Proc 1938;13:715–718.
Woolling KR. Wolfram syndrome: a tribute to Don J Wolfram MD. Indiana Medicine 1989 July;82(7):548–549.

Review and Case Reports:
Leiva-Santana C, Carro-Martinez A, Monge-Argiles A, Palao-Sanchez A. Neurologic manifestations in Wolfram's syndrome. Rev Neurol (Paris) 1993;149(1):26–29.
Domenech E, Gomez-Zaera M, Nunes V. Wolfram/DIDMOAD syndrome, a heterogenic and molecularly complex neurodegenerative disease. Pediatr Endocrinol Rev 2006 Mar;3(3): 249–257.

X

X-Linked Opitz G/BBB Syndrome

X-Linked Opitz G/BBB Syndrome

J.G. Millichap, *Neurological Syndromes: A Clinical Guide to Symptoms and Diagnosis*, DOI 10.1007/978-1-4614-7786-0_23,
© Springer Science+Business Media New York 2013

X-Linked Opitz G/BBB Syndrome
(alt: Opitz syndrome; XLOS)

- Organs Involved
  - Face, eyes, laryngotracheoesophageal, genitourinary, cerebellar vermis, corpus callosum

- Diagnostic Characteristics
  - Ocular hypertelorism
  - Hypospadias
  - Laryngotracheoesophageal abnormalities, cleft palate
  - Intellectual disability
  - Midline brain defects (corpus callosum and cerebellar vermis agenesis)
  - Congenital heart defects
  - Imperforate anus

- Genetics
  - X-linked inheritance, with mutations in the MID1 gene
  - Diagnosis suspected in males with ocular hypertelorism and at least one other major characteristic

References

Original:
Opitz JM, Summitt RL, Smith DW. The BBB syndrome familial telecanthus with associated congenital anomalies. Birth Defects: Original Article Series 1969b;2(V):86–94.

Review and Case Reports:
Ferrentino R, Basi MT, Chitayat D, Tabolacci E, Meroni G. MID1 mutation screening in a large cohort of Opitz G/BBB syndrome patients: twenty-nine novel mutations identified. Hum Mutat 2007;28:206–207.
Meroni G. X-linked Opitz G/BBB syndrome. In: Pagon RA, Bird TD, Dolan CR, et al., editors. GeneReviews [internet], Seattle (WA): University of Washington, Seattle;1993-Update July 28, 2011.

Z

Zellweger Syndrome

Zellweger Syndrome

J.G. Millichap, *Neurological Syndromes: A Clinical Guide to Symptoms and Diagnosis*, DOI 10.1007/978-1-4614-7786-0_24,
© Springer Science+Business Media New York 2013

Zellweger Syndrome
(alt: Cerebrohepatorenal syndrome)

- Organs Involved
  - Peroxisomes, brain, face, liver, kidney, cartilage, eye, hearing

- Diagnostic Abnormalities
  - A peroxisome biogenesis disorder
  - Impaired neuronal migration and brain development
  - Microgyria, polymicrogyria, pachygyria, leukoencephalopathy
  - Sensorineural degeneration with impaired hearing and vision
  - Eye abnormalities, cataracts
  - Craniofacial abnormalities (high forehead, midface hypoplasia)
  - Hepatomegaly, chondrodysplasia punctate
  - Cardiac complications, renal cysts

- Associated Abnormalities
  - Congenital hypotonia
  - Seizures

- Genetics
  - Autosomal recessive disorder caused by mutations in genes that encode peroxins (PEX1-26), resulting in reduction of peroxisomes in tissue cells
  - Accumulation of very long chain fatty acids (VLCFA) and branched chain fatty acids (BCFA) normally degraded in peroxisomes

- Prognosis
  - Life span of a few weeks or months

References

Original:
Bowen P, Lee CSN, Zellweger HU, Lindenburg R. A familial syndrome of multiple congenital defects. Bull Johns Hopkins Hospital 1964;114:402.
Opitz JM et al. The Zellweger syndrome (cerebro-hepato-renal syndrome). Birth Defects Original Article Series, New York 1969;5(2):144–160.

Review and Case Reports:
Weller S, Rosewich H, Gartner J. Cerebral MRI as a valuable diagnostic tool in Zellweger spectrum patients. J Inherit Metab Dis 2008 Apr;31(2):270–280.
Brul SWA, Westerveld A, Strijland A, et al. Genetic heterogeneity in the cerebrohepatorenal (Zellweger) syndrome and other inherited disorders with a generalized impairment of peroxisomal functions. A study using complementation analysis. Jrnl Clin Investigation 1988 Jun;81(6):1710–1715.

Index